Nutrition for Children

Dorothy E. M. Francis, SRD

Group Chief Dietitian
The Hospitals for Sick Children
Great Ormond Street, London

With a Foreword by

Barbara E. Clayton

CBE MD PhD DSc FRCP FRCPE PRCPath
Honorary Fellow of the British Dietetic Association
Dean of the Faculty of Medicine
and Professor of Chemical Pathology
and Human Metabolism
University of Southampton

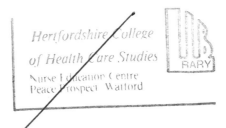

BLACKWELL SCIENTIFIC PUBLICATIONS
OXFORD LONDON EDINBURGH
BOSTON PALO ALTO MELBOURNE

©1986 by Blackwell Scientific
Publications
Editorial offices:
Osney Mead, Oxford OX2 0EL
8 John Street, London WC1N 2ES
23 Ainslie Place, Edinburgh EH3 6AJ
52 Beacon Street, Boston
    Massachusetts 02108, USA
667 Lytton Avenue, Palo Alto
    California 94301, USA
107 Barry Street, Carlton
    Victoria 3053, Australia

First published 1986

Typeset by Oxprint Ltd, Oxford

Printed and bound in Great Britain by
Billing and Sons Ltd, Worcester

DISTRIBUTORS

USA
    Blackwell Mosby Book Distributors
    11830 Westline Industrial Drive
    St Louis, Missouri 63141

Canada
    The C. V. Mosby Company
    5240 Finch Avenue East
    Scarborough, Ontario

Australia
    Blackwell Scientific Publications
    (Australia) Pty Ltd
    107 Barry Street
    Carlton, Victoria 3053

British Library
Cataloguing in Publication Data

Francis, Dorothy E.M.
    Nutrition for children.
    1. Children — Nutrition
    I. Title
    613.2′088054   RJ206

    ISBN 0-632-01478-4

Contents

Foreword

Nutrition has never been under more active discussion by the population generally than at the present time. There are tremendous gaps in our knowledge and it is all too easy to make claims which sound as though they are based on hard scientific facts. There is increasing evidence that nutrition in early life and during childhood has a profound effect on health in later life and is therefore important in the prevention of disease.

However, the advice offered to professional workers and parents is often conflicting and they feel confused.

Nutrition for Children is the first of two books replacing three editions of the previous *Diets for Sick Children*, which were published in 1965, 1970 and 1974 respectively. A fourth edition of *Diets for Sick Children* is to be published later in 1986, dealing with therapeutic diets. This development is a measure both of the complexity of the subject and of the importance now attached to the feeding of healthy infants and children as well as the treatment of the sick child.

I know of no one more fitted to produce this book than Miss Dorothy Francis. Such an authoritative, up-to-date work has been required for a long time.

Those of us privileged to work with Miss Francis know that we learn something new every time we have a conversation with her. In this book she brings to the subject not only a deep knowledge of the science of nutrition in health and disease, but her understanding of infants, children and their parents, her practical approach, and her common sense, pervade her writing, as always. It is a privilege to write this Foreword and I congratulate Miss Francis most warmly on her achievement in producing a book which, I believe, makes a major contribution to the care of the child.

Barbara E. Clayton

Preface

The past few years have seen a growing interest in nutrition in health and disease. A role for nutrition in the prevention of disease has been posed, and given wide media coverage. Many people are confused by conflicting and, in some cases, extreme opinions expressed which are not necessarily based on scientific fact.

Children are unique as optimal growth is of paramount importance for them, and the commonest nutritional disorder of the western world, namely overweight, is unusual before adolescence and affects only 5% of all children compared with 5 – 39% of adults. The purpose of this book is to detail the nutritional needs of infants and children to promote optimal growth avoiding extremes of both under- and over-nutrition. It provides parents and professionals with a practical guide for feeding children in the 1980s.

The special dietary regimens required for the treatment of disease are dealt with in my book *Diets for Sick Children*, published by Blackwell Scientific Publications. A largely rewritten and revised 4th edition is due for publication in 1986.

A number of specially prepared products such as infant formulae are available. The composition and ingredients of products change relatively frequently and vary from country to country. The export variety may differ from the product sold in the country of origin. Scoops included for reconstituting the product also differ and therefore only that supplied with the product and the manufacturer's instruction for preparation should be followed explicitly. The latest nutritional data should be obtained from the manufacturer. Although the latest product data has been checked during the preparation of this book, no responsibility can be taken for any product quoted and other similar products to those quoted may be equally suitable.

Dorothy E. M. Francis

Acknowledgements

I would like to acknowledge the encouragement and advice given to me in the preparation of this book by Professor Barbara Clayton, CBE, MD, PhD, DSc, FRCP, FRCPE, PRCPath, Dean of the Faculty of Medicine, University of Southampton. I am also grateful for advice given to me by Dr Olga Stark, MD, with the section on overweight and obesity, Dr Peter Milla, MSc, MBBS, MRCP regarding the section on catabolism and Dr Peter Aggett, MSc, MB, ChB, MRCP, MRCS, LRCP, DCH for assistance with the section on trace minerals. I would also like to thank Rebecca Knowles and Elisabeth Moore for secretarial help with this book.

Introduction

Any diet must be both nutritionally adequate for growth and acceptable socially and financially.

Recommended daily intakes and safe and adequate ranges quoted are intended for population groups, and diets based on these require modification for the individual. The sample diets given in this book are intended as a guide, and must be adapted for the age and weight of an individual child and for nutrient intake, consistency and quantity.

Calculations are based on figures from *McCance & Widdowson's The Composition of Foods* (Paul & Southgate 1978) and manufacturers' data on special products. Metrication and SI units are now accepted in the United Kingdom, and used throughout with appropriate alternatives such as kilocalorie (kcal). Kilojoules (kJ) are used as a more appropriate measure of energy than megajoules (mJ) for paediatric diets. Conversion factors are given in Appendices 2 and 3.

A diet for use in the home should be described in practical household terms and measures such as calibrated scoops, teaspoons or tablespoons (Cameron & Hofvander 1983) unless weighing of food is essential. A demonstration showing the correct measurement of ingredients, feed making and special cooking is helpful if an unfamiliar item is advised, e.g., home preparation of infant weaning foods is unfamiliar to many first time mothers.

BASIC PRINCIPLES FOR DIET AND MENU PLANNING

Acceptability

In constructing diets it is necessary to consider religious and racial habits as well as individual likes and dislikes. It is important to consider the following aspects which should preface the details of any diet.

1

Palatability

The average child is suspicious of any food which is unfamiliar. New flavours and new kinds of food should be introduced with care, and, when possible, with other foods which are familiar. A choice of food should be offered to allow freedom of taste, and development of normal food habits. Savoury foods have grown in popularity and some racial groups include highly spiced foods from an early age without ill effect.

Appearance and Texture

The diet should look attractive and appeal to the visual appreciation of the child. Careful attention to garnishing the food with contrasting coloured vegetables and fruits will give pleasure even to a small patient. Texture of food is important: purées, milk puddings and cream soups should be smooth, and crisp food should be crunchy. Green vegetables should not be over-cooked but will need to be finely chopped for very young children; root vegetables should be diced, sliced or mashed. Meat should be cooked and finely minced or chopped for the toddler; for the pre-school child meat can be cut up into bite size pieces which are easy to chew; fish can be flaked with a fork for young children.

Serving of Food

Meals should be served at regular times. The interval between meals will vary with the age of the child, and if the child is unwell the nature and type of illness, but the spacing should be arranged to allow for the process of digestion and normally for uninterrupted sleep during the night. Young or sick children often benefit from several snacks in addition to the traditional meal times. Supplements may be needed to ensure adequate energy in children with poor appetites or during or immediately after a period of illness to promote nutritional repletion, provided appetite is not further suppressed by the supplement.

Small quantities served on dishes not larger than necessary are preferable; a second helping may be given if desired. Individual portions of cold sweets and jellies are more attractive than those prepared in bulk.

Utensils for the Child

The attractive coloured ware now seen in stores is appreciated by children and should be used instead of plain white ware. Unbreakable plastic ware is recommended. It must withstand the cleaning and sterilizing procedures needed in hospitals. Plates with deep edges and cereal bowls are better for the young child, who tends to scatter food around. Short-handled spoons with shallow bowls are recommended, as they fit the hands of a small child better than dessert spoons. Mugs and cups are easier than glasses for a small child to hold, and 'teacher beakers' are ideal during the weaning stage. Drinking straws are often useful in encouraging older children to drink and preventing spillage of fluids, and are of particular use for the sick child, after an operation and for unfamiliar or unpalatable drinks, e.g., soya milk substitutes.

Psycho-social Aspects

Most pre-school children go through a period of food refusal. This problem is usually short-lived and best ignored (Burman 1982). Parents need reassurance that the well child will not come to harm even if the diet is temporarily bizarre or inadequate (Bentovim 1970). Acceptable alternative foods and snacks can be offered and the child permitted to self-select the dietary intake according to appetite. The parents should be encouraged to ignore food refusal, otherwise meals can become a battleground and even child abuse may result. Force-feeding should be avoided. Social eating with a peer group at a nursery or school should be encouraged.

In persistent refusal or where there is failure to thrive a detailed 24-hour diet history and an estimation of the offered and consumed dietary intake may highlight the problem. Appropriate advice and help should be provided regarding the diet and handling of the child. A praise and reward system is often successful in achieving acceptance of essential items required for the child's health. Further investigation to rule out organic disease must be pursued if the situation does not improve or if it is warranted by the clinical condition.

Food refusal, or over-indulgence, is more common where the mother-child bonding has not been firmly established in infancy. Parental anxiety is increased by a poor appetite associated with intercurrent infection or chronic illness where the child's future is of major concern.

Diets and treatment necessitated by chronic illness in which cultural eating habits may be changed, increase the risk of feeding difficulties (Smith & Francis 1982). The seriousness of the illness and necessity to comply with a diet increases parental anxiety and depression can be a feature. Any diet limitations, stress of being different and social implications all play a part in the feeding difficulties. The parents should be provided with a list of priorities and usually energy intake is of primary importance. Instructions regarding adequate and acceptable energy sources should be given (Francis 1979). In dealing with feeding problems the anxiety of those supervising management should not be directed at the parents who are already under pressure. Critical comments and reprimands are almost always out of place. One approach to the management of the 'difficult' toddler on a therapeutic diet has been described by Smith *et al.* (1975). On rare occasions when the dietary intake is leading to serious malnutrition, at a time in the child's life when inadequate growth is likely to cause serious or long-term harm, management and parental support as frequently used in cases of child abuse is appropriate. In general, however, parental imperfections and occasional failures must be accepted with good grace.

Anorexia nervosa which usually occurs in the young female adult or teenager is a complex phenomenon resulting in severe malnutrition and requires management by an experienced team (Horder 1978; Norton 1983). It can occasionally co-exist with other chronic disorders such as diabetes mellitis (Belton & Farquhar 1984).

Diet and Dental Disease

There has been a reduction in dental caries recently reported (Infirri 1984) and this is attributed to the use of fluoride toothpaste and oral hygiene rather than dietary change. Sucrose has however been implicated as a major factor in the incidence of dental caries (King 1978), but an adequate energy intake is required for growth in children. Frequency of carbohydrate intake is also important. Glucose syrups at least in rats (Grenby & Leer 1974) and starches are less caries-inducing than sucrose. Other factors of importance in the formation of the teeth and which influence the occurrence of caries should be borne in mind, e.g., hereditary, neonatal hypocalcaemia (Stimmler *et al.* 1973), fluoride intake and dietary nutrients such as calcium, phosphorous and vitamin D both during fetal development and in the child's diet. Adequate oral hygiene with plaque removal reduces the incidence of caries (Winter & Murray 1974).

REFERENCES

BELTON N. R. & FARQUHAR, J. W. (1984) Diabetes mellitus. In Clayton B. E. & Round J. M. (eds) *Chemical Pathology and the Sick Child*, pp.265–95. Blackwell Scientific Publications, Oxford.

BENTOVIM A. (1970) The clinical approach to feeding disorders of childhood. *Journal of Psychosomatic Research* **14**, 267.

BURMAN D. (1982) Nutrition in early childhood. In McLaren D. S. & Burman D. (eds) *Textbook of Paediatric Nutrition*, 2nd ed., pp.39–73. Churchill Livingstone, Edinburgh.

CAMERON M. & HOFVANDER Y. (1983) *Manual on Feeding Infants and Young Children*, 3rd ed. Protein-Calorie Advisory Group of the United Nations System, United Nations, New York. Oxford University Press, Oxford.

FRANCIS D. E. M. (1979) Inborn errors of metabolism—the need for sugar. *The Journal of Human Nutrition* **33**, 146–54.

GRENBY T. H. & LEER C. J. (1974) Reduction in 'smooth-surface' caries and fat accumulation in rats when sucrose in drinking water is replaced by glucose syrup. *Caries Research* **8**, 368–72.

HORDER D.M. (1978) Anorexia nervosa—do we recognise it? *Nutrition Bulletin* **4**, 304–13.

INFIRRI J. (1984) Trends in the patterns of oral disease: implications for Ireland. *Journal of the Irish Dental Association,* **April/June,** 13–19.

KING J. M. (1978) Patterns of sugar consumption in early infancy. *Community Dentistry Oral Epidemiology* **6**, 46–52.

NORTON K. (1983) Anorexia Nervosa. *Midwife, Health Visitor and Community Nurse* **19**, 310–14.

PAUL A. A. & SOUTHGATE D. A. T. (1978) *McCance and Widdowson's The Composition of Foods*, 4th revised ed. HMSO, London.

SMITH I., FRANCIS D. E. M., CLAYTON B. E. & WOLFF O. H. (1975) Comparison of an amino acid mixture and protein hydrolysate in treatment of infants with phenylketonuria. *Archives of Disease in Childhood* **50,** 864.

SMITH I. & FRANCIS D. E. M. (1982) Disorders of amino acid metabolism. In McLaren D. S. & Burman D. (eds) *Textbook of Paediatric Nutrition*, 2nd ed., pp.295–323. Churchill Livingstone, Edinburgh.

STIMMLER I., SNODGRASS G. J. A. & JAFFE E. (1973) Dental defects associated with neonatal symptomatic hypocalcaemia. *Archives of Disease in Childhood* **48**, 217–20.

WINTER G. B. & MURRAY J. J. (1974) Dental caries: its causes, prevention and control. In Harty F. J. & Roberts D. H. (eds) *Dental Caries*, pp.71–90. John Wright & Sons, Bristol.

CHAPTER 1

Nutrition in Health and Disease

Children differ from adults because their nutritional intake must provide not only for the replacement of tissues but also for growth. The *Textbook of Paediatric Nutrition*, 2nd ed., edited by McLaren & Burman (1982) reviews the role of nutrition in childhood, maternal nutrition and fetal growth, and nutritional disorders. The nutritional adequacy of any diet is determined by the clinical state, growth and development of the child. The energy and nutritional needs can be achieved by widely differing food and meal patterns, though nutrient density is important for the young child to prevent the problems of under- and over-nutrition associated with the bulk of food needed to provide the nutritional needs (Cameron & Hofvander 1983). Nutritional problems are most likely to occur in infancy and adolescence during periods of rapid growth, and are frequently related to infections and catabolic states. The sick child is therefore at greatest risk of growth failure and nutritional disorders.

Fetal growth is important in determining the birth weight of the infant and at least in part is related to the mother's diet, state of health and height, as well as the gestational age of the infant at birth. The maximum velocity of fetal growth appears to be between 32 and 38 weeks of gestation during which interval the weight virtually doubles (Metcoff 1982). Gestational age and birth weight of the infant largely determine the ability of the infant to adapt to extra-uterine life.

Normal birth weight for infants under optimal conditions varies between 3.3 and 3.5 kg in both sexes. Low birth weight is defined as being below 2.5 kg and those below 1.5 kg are known as very low birth weight. This may be due to either short gestation (premature, i.e., less than 37 weeks gestation) or retarded fetal growth (small for dates) related to maternal nutrition and environmental factors including placental function (Metcoff 1982). Such infants have special nutritional needs in the first months of life though there is debate as to what is optimal (DHSS 1981; Brooke *et al.* 1982; Burman 1982). Breast-feeding is strongly recommended for the full-term infant in the first months of life (DHSS 1983, revised) and few would disagree with this recommendation.

Weight increases rapidly in the first months of life, usually doubling the birth weight in 3 to 5 months and it trebles in the first year of life and length increases by 50%. Table 1.1 gives a guide to the expected weight and height gain during the first 2 years of life. There is a rapid change in the ratio of surface area to weight or height. Catzel (1974) expresses this as a percentage of adult surface area, and Butler & Richie (1960) suggested nutritional requirements are better expressed in relationship to surface area rather than weight or height. However for the purposes of monitoring growth, measurement of height and weight are normally appropriate. Nutritional requirements are often expressed according to weight. Height and weight percentile charts give the range of weight and height for children of different ages (Tanner & Whitehouse 1976) and are an excellent comparison for the growth of an individual child if a series of measurements are available over a period of time. Growth charts for international use are available from the World Health Organization (WHO 1978). Growth velocity charts are also available (Tanner & Whitehouse 1976). Arm circumference measurements (Cameron & Hofvander 1983), and skinfold measurements are useful in assessing under- and over-nutrition. McLaren (1982a) lists these and other anthropometric measurements together with useful signs and biochemical tests used in assessing nutritional status.

NUTRIENT REQUIREMENTS

Recommendations for nutritional intake of population groups of

Table 1.1 Expected gain in weight and height in infants.

Weight	Height
200 g (7 oz) per week for the first 3 months 150 g (≈5 oz) per week for the second 3 months 100 g (3½ oz) per week for the third 3 months 50–75 g (1¾–2¾ oz) per week in the fourth 3 months	Approximately 25 cm (10 inches) in length during the first year
2.5 kg (5½ lb) weight gain during the second year	Approximately 12 cm (5 inches) in length during the second year

healthy people have been given by a number of organizations (WHO 1974; DHSS 1985; NRC 1980). Table 1.2 is adapted from this information. Guidelines for the safe range of micromineral intakes are summarized from Aggett & Davies (1983) (Table 3.5). Recommended intakes vary in different reports and as more knowledge becomes available. The figures relate to population groups and are not intended to be related to an individual. The recommendation for any one nutrient presupposes adequacy of all other nutrients. For children allowance is made for the needs of normal growth. It has been estimated that 20 kJ (5 kcal) is needed for each gram of body weight gain in growth. Approximately one quarter to one third of the energy intake in the first months of life is used for growth. The optimal intake for an individual is that which satisfies needs and allows for normal growth and activity. In many instances, excess is of no importance but in a few instances it may be harmful, e.g., excess vitamin D can cause hypercalcaemia.

Requirements differ from one individual to another by ± 15% and change with alteration in the composition and nature of the diet because such alteration affects the efficiency with which nutrients are absorbed and utilized. For example, phytate commonly associated with fibre in foods can inhibit the availability of calcium and zinc. This is particularly important in largely cereal-based diets such as fruitarian and Zen macrobiotic diets which are not recommended for children as they provide inadequate nutrition for optimal growth.

The recommendations do not cover additional needs arising from disease, for catch-up growth, malabsorption or metabolic abnormalities. Catabolism particularly increases the requirement of nutrients (pp.59–79).

Apart from the nutrients listed, all other nutrients including trace elements and vitamins (see Chapter 3) must be supplied. The requirements of some of the trace elements are less well established but are usually supplied from a diet based on a wide variety of foods which covers the requirement of the nutrients listed. Restricted and synthetic diets however necessitate particular attention to all nutrients.

Protein

Protein is a source not only of energy but of nitrogen in the body which is an essential part of all tissues, cells and enzymes. Protein requirement must be considered in conjunction with energy needs because unless it is fully met protein will be used as energy instead of being available for essential functions and growth. This is particularly important in low protein diets used, e.g., in renal and liver disease. Growth failure is frequently a consequence of protein energy malnutrition and can occur when protein intake is restricted. Protein needs are at a maximum during periods of rapid growth in infancy and childhood, during infections and injury.

Proteins are made from a mixture of about 22 amino acids in varying proportions. The amino group NH_2 cannot be synthesized by man. Eight amino acids plus histidine in children are essential and must be provided in the diet. Several additional amino acids are considered semi-essential in infants in whom enzymes necessary for amino acid metabolism are immature. These include cystine, tyrosine, arginine and possibly proline and glycine. Provided adequate nitrogen is available the non-essential amino acids can be synthesized in the body.

There is an ideal pattern of the essential amino acids for human protein synthesis and this is known as reference protein (WHO 1974). A food protein in which the amino acids pattern closely resembles this pattern can be completely used for protein synthesis in the body, i.e., the net protein utilization (NPU) = 100 and closely resembles the protein score calculated from the limiting amino acid (Burman 1982). Egg and human milk closely resemble the reference protein pattern and have an NPU or score of 100. Cereals, legumes and vegetable proteins are limited in one or more essential amino acids and have a lower NPU and diets based on these foods may only have an NPU or score of 50 to 60 and therefore larger quantities of protein must be supplied in the diet for growth and protein synthesis. However, where different protein foods are eaten at the same meal their amino acid composition can complement each other, e.g., cereals low in lysine can be complemented by legumes which are rich in lysine but low in cystine and methionine; together better utilization of the amino acids can be made for protein synthesis.

The requirement of reference protein (NPU 100) assumes all the protein can be used for protein synthesis and therefore the requirement is less than from a mixed diet of animal and cereal protein (NPU 70 to 80) or a vegetarian diet (NPU 60 to 65) or a cereal-based diet, e.g., Zen macrobiotic diets (NPU 50). The requirement of protein given in Table 1.2 is based on 10% energy needs coming from protein with an NPU value of 75 (DHSS 1979). Most children in the industrialized world have an uptake of protein in excess of recommended intakes, and except in young infants and

Table 1.2 Recommended daily amounts of food energy and some nutrients for population groups in the United Kingdom. (Adapted from DHSS 1985 revision, NRC 1980 and WHO 1974.)

Age range[e]	Average expected body weight kg	Fluid ml/day for a full fluid diet[f]	Energy mean[ae] kJ	Energy mean[ae] kcal	Protein g[ag]	Thiamin mg[a]	Riboflavin mg[a]
Infants							
0–6 months		150[d]	490[cd]	117[cd]	2.2[cd]	0.3	0.4
6–12 months		150[d]	450[cd]	108[cd]	2.0[cd]	0.3	0.4
Boys							
1	11.5	1100	5000	1200	30.0	0.5	0.6
2	13.5	1300	5750	1400	35.0	0.6	0.7
3–4	16.5	1500	6500	1560	39.0	0.6	0.8
5–6	20.0	1700	7250	1740	43.0	0.7	0.9
7–8	25.0	1800	8250	1980	49.0	0.8	1.0
9–11	32.0	2200	9500	2280	57.0	0.9	1.2
12–14	44.0	2300	11 000	2640	66.0	1.1	1.4
15–17	62.0	3000	12 000	2880	72.0	1.2	1.7
Girls							
1	11.0	1050	4500	1100	27.0	0.4	0.6
2	13.5	1300	5500	1300	32.0	0.5	0.7
3–4	16.0	1450	6250	1500	37.0	0.6	0.8
5–6	20.0	1700	7000	1680	42.0	0.7	0.9
7–8	25.0	1800	8000	1900	47.0	0.8	1.0
9–11	32.0	2000	8500	2050	51.0	0.8	1.2
12–14	50.0	2200	9000	2150	53.0	0.9	1.4
15–17	56.0	2200	9000	2150	53.0	0.9	1.7

[a] DHSS 1985 revision. The average amount of a nutrient which should be provided per head in a group of people if the needs of practically all members of the group are to be met. Except for energy the recommended amounts represent a judgement of the average requirement plus a margin of safety.

[b] From NRC 1980.

[c] From WHO 1974.

[d] Value/kg actual body weight per day.

[e] Since the recommendations are average amounts, the figures for each age range represent the amounts recommended at the middle of the range. Within each age range, younger children will need less, and older children more, than the recommended amount.

[f] Suggested fluid intake for fluid and enteral feeds. Except in infants 1 ml = 1 kcal = 4.2 kJ is usually found satisfactory.

Nicotinic acid equivalents mg[ah]	B[12] µg[b]	Ascorbic acid vit. C mg[a]	Vitamin A retinal equivalents µg[ai]	Vitamin D chole calciferol µg[aj]	Calcium mmol[a]	Phosphorus mmol[b]	Iron mmol[a]
5	0.3	20	450	7.5	15.0	7.7	0.11
5	0.3	20	450	7.5	15.0	11.6	0.11
7	0.9	20	300	10.0	15.0	25.8	0.13
8	0.9	20	300	10.0	15.0	25.8	0.13
9	0.9	20	300	10.0	15.0	25.8	0.14
10	1.5	20	300	i	15.0	25.8	0.18
11	1.5	20	400	i	15.0	25.8	0.18
14	2.0	25	575	i	17.5	38.7	0.22
16	2.0	25	725	i	17.5	38.7	0.22
19	2.0	30	750	i	15.0	38.7	0.22
7	0.9	20	300	10.0	15.0	25.8	0.13
8	0.9	20	300	10.0	15.0	25.8	0.13
9	0.9	20	300	10.0	15.0	25.8	0.14
10	1.5	20	300	i	15.0	25.8	0.18
11	1.5	20	400	i	15.0	25.8	0.18
14	2.0	25	575	i	17.5	38.7	0.22[k]
16	2.0	25	725	i	17.5	38.7	0.22[k]
19	2.0	30	750	i	17.5	38.7	0.22[k]

[g] Recommended amounts have been calculated as 10% of the recommendations for energy, except where sole source protein is from human milk.

[h] 1 nicotinic acid equivalent = 1 mg available nicotinic acid or 60 mg tryptophan.

[i] 1 retinol equivalent = 1 µg retinol or 6 µg β-carotene or 12 µg other biologically active carotenoids.

[j] No dietary sources may be necessary for children and adults who are sufficiently exposed to sunlight, but during the winter children and adolescents should receive 10 µg (400 i.u) daily by supplementation. Those with inadequate exposure to sunlight, for example those who are 'housebound' may also need a supplement of 10 µg daily.

[k] This intake may not be sufficient for 10% of girls with large menstrual loss.

[l] Guidelines for the safe range of micromineral intakes are summarised from Aggett & Davies 1983 (see Table 3.5).

those with chronic renal failure there is no indication that a moderate excess of protein is harmful for the normal population. Children on dietary regimens excluding first-class protein should be encouraged to have a generous protein intake and to include food combinations of cereals and legumes, e.g., beans on toast, to ensure adequate protein for growth. Minimum protein intakes should ideally be largely derived from high biological proteins with an NPU score of approximately 100. Infants receiving human milk can maintain growth on 1.8 g protein/kg per day in the first months of life and less by 6 months of age and adults can maintain nitrogen equilibrium on 0.35 to 0.45 g milk protein/kg per day providing energy and all other nutrient intake is adequate.

Utilization of protein for growth cannot occur unless adequate energy is provided. Likewise as the concentration of protein increases in the diet, the proportion used for body-building decreases; the remaining protein is used as energy. The percentage of energy from protein is a way of relating the two. Young infants up to the age of 6 months should as far as possible be breast-fed. Artificial milks and mixed diets should normally provide at least 10% of the energy as protein.

Energy (kilojoule/kilocalorie)

The recommendations for energy needs are based on averages for population groups. The intake for each individual must supply the need for energy expenditure and growth and will depend on age, sex and physical activity. Inevitably males grow more rapidly and consume higher energy intakes than females from early infancy onwards.

Under- and over-nutrition are the two major nutritional diseases and both are related to energy intake. Frequently energy density is a major factor (Burkitt et al. 1980). The high bulk, high fibre, lower energy content of available food in many third world countries leads to inadequate intake as small children can only take a certain maximum volume of 200 to 300 ml of food at any one time. This is a major factor in protein-energy malnutrition.

In a young child, who needs a high energy intake in relation to body weight, a high energy density is essential for normal growth. If fat intake is reduced and if in addition refined carbohydrates are avoided as recommended (James 1983; DHSS 1984) it will be difficult to achieve the necessary energy intake, at least in some young children. In order to ensure adequate energy intake with only 3 meals a day a content of 6 to 8.5 kJ (1.5 to 2 kcal) per g or ml of food is needed (Cameron & Hofvander 1983) or more meals and snacks are required. In the UK and Western world over-nutrition due to excess energy intake is the more common problem and high energy density expecially from refined carbohydrate and fat are contributory factors which can lead to obesity.

Individual requirements of energy vary widely from group recommendations. Recently Whitehead *et al.* (1981) has queried the validity of the FAO/WHO 1973 energy recommendations for growing healthy infants by comparing these with actual intakes from various studies both in the UK and other Western world countries. Particularly in infants aged 3 to 9 months the actual intakes, allowing for age and sex differences, were below the recommendations. The significance of this finding is still not clearly defined, but suggests earlier recommendations may be over generous. McKillop & Durnin (1982) in their survey of 305 children aged 3 months to 2 years, living in Glasgow, also found the intakes of protein and energy were lower than the DHSS (1979) recommended amounts though no evidence of malnutrition was detected. There was almost no variation due to social group, except the most favoured groups had the lowest energy intake and males had higher intakes than females. These surveys support the suggestion made by the DHSS (1979) recommendations that young children eat less than previously, but even these 1979 recommendations may still be set too high, even though they are lower than those suggested in 1969.

The nutrient content of different foods is available in *McCance & Widdowson's The Composition of Foods* (Paul & Southgate 1978) and many manufacturers will provide details of their products, so that dietary intakes can be calculated. The energy value of food is derived from protein, fat and carbohydrate. Conversion factors are given in Appendix 2. The energy distribution from these nutrients varies in different types of traditional diets and meal patterns.

For the majority of normal children a self-selected energy intake is appropriate and achieves satisfactory growth. Modification by education on food priorities to encourage better nutrition may be necessary. Force-feeding and concentrated energy supplements are not normally advised. However many young children benefit from 3 meals and 2 to 3 snacks per day to ensure adequate opportunity to eat an appropriate intake. Children with a tendency to obesity are better advised to have only 3 meals per day.

Fat

Fats are essential to provide adequate energy, essential fatty acid and fat-soluble vitamins. Fat is also important in making food palatable.

Essential fatty acid deficiency in infants (Hansen *et al*. 1962) leads to growth retardation, skin changes with hair loss, increased metabolic rate and even early death. Linoleic acid C18:2 n-6 and possibly α-linolenic acid C18:3 n-3 are the only essential fatty acids (DHSS 1980a). Linoleic acid should provide at least 1.2% energy (DHSS 1979), and FAO/WHO (1980) recommends 3% energy from essential fatty acids for normal infants and adults. Infants may have a higher requirement in order to permit optimal neural development (Crawford *et al*. 1976), though deficiency has not been observed in infants fed on cow's milk fat formulae (Naismith *et al*. 1978). The DHSS (1980a) suggest a limit for polyunsaturated fatty acids in infant feeds of a maximum of 16 to 20% of total fatty acid.

Fat is normally well absorbed (approximately 97%) in children, but infants cannot absorb certain fatty acids very efficiently. Barltrop (1974) showed the retention of different fatty acids from butterfat in infants varied inversely with the number of carbons and the unsaturated fatty acids were better absorbed (Table 1.3). Butterfat is therefore not ideal for infant nutrition as it is poorly absorbed and is low in essential fatty acid content, containing only 0.5% energy from linoleic acid C18:2. Human milk fat has a higher proportion of mono-unsaturated fatty acids and polyunsaturated fatty acids but linoleic acid C18:2 varies from 1 to 15% energy

Table 1.3 Retention of individual fatty acids from butterfat by infants. (From Barltrop 1974.)

Fatty acid		Retention %
Caprylic	$C_{8:0}$	100
Capric	$C_{10:0}$	100
Lauric	$C_{12:0}$	83
Myristic	$C_{14:0}$	67
Palmitic	$C_{16:0}$	46
Palmitoleic	$C_{16:1}$	69
Stearic	$C_{18:0}$	29
Oleic	$C_{18:1}$	63
Linoleic	$C_{18:2}$	78
Linolenic	$C_{18:3}$	80

depending on the maternal diet (DHSS 1980a). Human milk fat is better absorbed: 90% at 1 week old compared to only 70% of butterfat and an intermediate figure for milks containing a mixture of animal and vegetable fats. This is related to the type of fatty acids, their position on the glycerol molecule and lipase content of human milk which enhances absorption.

The higher incidence of heart disease in the Western world is multifactorial and includes such factors as obesity, diabetes, smoking, hypertension, lack of exercise and stress, as well as possibly diet. The debate about dietary fat and coronary heart disease (CHD) is complex and controversial (James 1983; Oliver 1984; Lancet, Editorials 1984a,b; DHSS 1984; Mitchell 1984; Moore 1984).

Various reports (Passmore et al. 1979; James 1983; DHSS 1984) have suggested a decrease in dietary fat in the hope of reducing the incidence of CHD in the population as a whole. The latter report recommends a reduction in saturated fat, inclusive of trans fats, to 15% dietary energy and total fat to 35% energy intake with a polyunsaturated to saturated fatty acid (P/S) ratio of 0.45. These recommendations are based on (i) the lipid hypothesis, that is a high dietary fat intake causes a high blood cholesterol and this increases the risk of CHD and (ii) epidemiology studies relating population dietary fat intakes with the incidence of CHD. However, these studies do not take into account genetic factors related to cholesterol metabolism, or the individual response which occurs as a result of dietary change in quantity and type of fat (Ahrens 1979). The Committee on Medical Aspects (COMA) of Food Policy Report of the Panel on Diet in Relation to Cardiovascular Disease (DHSS 1984) in its consideration of the complex relationship between diet and CHD, has acknowledged that the evidence falls short of proof and their recommendations for the general public are a majority decision of 9 out of 10 members though all agree they should be advised for people with an increased risk of CHD.

The recommendations for dietary change (DHSS 1984) are addressed to the general public as a whole and not to subgroups or individuals within the populace and 'are intended mainly for older children and young and middle-aged adults. . . . They are not intended for infants (i.e., those under one year of age) and the recommendation for fat is not appropriate for children under the age of five.' The latter is on the advice from the Panel of Child Nutrition of the Committee on Medical Aspects of Food Policy relating to 'children below the age of five who usually obtain a substantial proportion of dietary energy from cow's milk.' The report also states 'Families who elect to switch from whole cow's milk to semi-skimmed or skimmed milk in implementing the recommendations for fat, are advised in the light of current evidence to continue to provide whole cow's milk for children below the age of five.'

Any alteration to the composition of the diet has profound effects on the intake of other nutrients and must be carefully assessed before it is generally implemented, particularly in young children. If a reduction of fat is appropriate, nutritionally acceptable alternative physiological sources of the energy lost are essential except in those who are overweight and care must be taken to provide essential fatty acids and fat-soluble vitamins needed for healthy development.

Milk is a major constituent in the diet of infants and young children. Infants should be breast-fed or given a modified whey-based infant formula (Tables 1.5 & 1.6). A child of 2 years who is taking 500 ml whole milk in the diet per day obtains in terms of nutrient recommended intakes, approximately 50% protein, 24% energy, 64% vitamin A and 100% of both calcium and riboflavin. To reduce the fat content of the whole diet, an apparently simple measure would appear to be to use skimmed milk. There is no proof either that milk fat is harmful to children or that its substitution by other items in the diet would be beneficial. Skimmed milk has a much lower energy density so that 500 ml provides only 12% of the energy needs of a 2-year-old and almost no fat-soluble vitamins or essential fatty acids. Skimmed milk like whole milk and goat's milk has the disadvantage of too high a protein, sodium and renal solute making them unsuitable for young infants (DHSS 1983, revised; Yeung et al. 1982) or as the sole source of nutrition.

In the Canadian study by Yeung et al. (1982) the nutrient intake of children during the first year taking 2% fat milk (semi-skimmed milk) had similar growth and energy intakes compared to the infants taking whole fat milk. The fat intake of the total diet was reduced in those on the 2% fat milk (24 to 29% energy from fat). However, in order to compensate the reduced fat intake contributed from fat, additional milk was taken and they tended to eat more food with the result that higher protein, sodium, renal solute, calcium, phosphorus and potassium were taken. The higher protein (18 to 20% energy intake) and higher renal solute loads that resulted were considered inappropriate because of the potential risk of pre-renal azotema and hyperosmolar state, even though they did not adversely affect growth. The relatively low level of fat in the 2% fat milk may also be undesirable because of the potential risk of inadequate essential fatty acid intake if other foods do not compensate the deficit. Thus, skimmed milk and semi-skimmed milks should not be recommended generally for children under 5 years old and if used should only be in conjunction with a nutritionally adequate diet. Milk plays a diminishing nutritional role from school age and therefore it is optional whether skimmed milk, reduced fat or whole milk is used in the diet of the older child, who can more easily obtain the energy deficit from other foods.

In the study of the nutrient intake of 4-year-old Australian children (Magarey & Boulton 1984) the children were eating less than recommended intakes of energy but were growing normally. They ate less from main food groups compared to children reported in other studies but the contribution to daily energy intake was comparable, except for an increased protein (mean 14% energy with a range of 10 to 20%) which compensated for a lower fat (mean 35% energy with a range of 25 to 45%). A relatively high intake of refined carbohydrates as sweets and sweetened drinks were also reported. In general the lower fat intake did not lead to an overall improvement in nutrition as the higher protein intake is an inappropriate way to compensate the energy deficit from fat, as is an overall high sugar and refined carbohydrate.

Vegetable oils which are higher in polyunsaturated fatty acids such as soya, safflower, sunflower, corn and to a lesser extent olive oil may be preferable to hard fats and other vegetable oils. Their use in the diet as a replacement of other fats will help increase the polyunsaturated:saturated fatty acid (P/S) ratio of the diet to the recommended 0.45. However, excessive use of polyunsaturated fatty acids, providing a diet with a P/S ratio in excess of 1, is *not* recommended (DHSS 1984). Repeated heating of oils during cooking hydrogenates some of the unsaturated fatty acids. Also the hydrogenation process used in the manufacture of margarine not only produces saturated fatty acids but *trans* fatty acids which are not present to any extent in traditional fat sources (Thomas *et al.* 1981; Kochhar & Matsui 1984). The latter provides analysis data on different fat sources in the UK. This shows that margarines based on fish oils have the highest *trans* fatty acid content (21 to 42%) whereas the polyunsaturated margarines based on vegetable oils had a lower *trans* fatty acid content. Although butterfat was low in polyunsaturated fatty acids, it also had a low *trans* fatty acid content. Until further work establishes the safety of *trans* fatty acids, which are currently thought to act similarly to saturated fatty acids in human metabolism (Thomas *et al.* 1981), margarines high in *trans* fatty acids cannot be recommended without some reservation, at least for children's diets. Those who elect to use a margarine should be advised to use a polyunsaturated margarine derived solely from vegetable oils.

A modest reduction in total fat intake may be appropriate, but the energy contribution from fat will vary with age and circumstances of the individual. Those identified as having familial hypercholesterolaemia (Francis in press) should be advised to limit more rigorously their fat intake after the first year of life. Fat intake should be reduced by using lean meat and reserving fried foods, crisps, etc. to occasional rather than every day items.

Fibre

Dietary fibre is useful in increasing faecal output and prevention of constipation. A number of diseases associated with Western industrialized society have been correlated with a lack of dietary fibre (Burkitt *et al.* 1980). Wholegrain cereals, fruit and vegetables as well as providing dietary fibre contribute other nutrients, minerals and vitamins to the diet. However, phytate which is commonly associated with dietary fibre present in cereals and pulses, inhibits the absorption of certain minerals (Aggett & Davies 1983) although wholegrain cereals contain higher quantities of calcium, iron and zinc compared to refined cereals. Bran supplements added to a refined cereal diet is less desirable than a wholegrain cereal-based diet; unprocessed bran to increase fibre is not recommended in young children, especially under 2 years of age. Wholegrain cereals and wholemeal bread can be introduced into the diet gradually from about 8 months when finger foods are introduced into the weaning regimen. Wholemeal bread is a particularly useful source of dietary fibre as the phytase in yeast destroys phytate. The National Advisory Committee on Nutrition Education (NACNE) recommendations (James 1983) for dietary fibre to be increased to 23 g per day initially and 30 g per day ultimately are inappropriate for children as fibre intake must be proportional to energy requirements. A careful balance between fibre intake and energy density is necessary to avoid the extremes of under- and over-nutrition. Intakes of dietary fibre are not established for children.

NEWBORN INFANTS

Breast-feeding is a major preventive medicine measure which markedly reduces infant mortality and disease (Ebrahim 1978; Jelliffe & Jelliffe 1978). It is possible in every village of the world. The decline in breast-feeding of the 1960s and early 1970s has been largely due to lack of interest by the professionals and inappropriate milk marketing practice (Chetley 1979). The incidence of breast-feeding in England and Wales has gradually increased recently (Martin & Monk 1982).

Appropriate nutrition for growth and development is essential to the child's well-being and subsequent development. Human milk is designed to meet the changing nutritional needs of the young infant and exclusive demand breast-feeding is recommended for the first 4 to 6 months of life, with appropriate vitamins (p.42) and the introduction of weaning solids (pp.42–5) normally from 4 months and not usually later than 6 months.

Recently, several reports on infant feeding have been published setting guidelines and recommendations such as *Present Day Practice in Infant Feeding* (DHSS 1983, revised), and *Artificial Feeds for the Young Infant* (DHSS 1980a). The 1980 survey into infant feeding practice in England, Wales and Scotland (Martin & Monk 1982) highlights the shortfall from the 1974 recommendations that infants should be breast-fed, and solids delayed until 4 months. Although more infants are initially breast-fed in 1980 (67%) than in 1975 (51%) very few are breast-fed for the minimum length of time, 4 months, that is recommended. Breast-feeding failure frequently occurs in the first 2 weeks of life. The survey highlights a number of influencing factors on breast-feeding failure and choice of infant feeding including social class, mothers' education, birth order of the infant, birth experience of mother and her baby together. The technique and feeding practice in the hospital, delay from the time of birth to first suckling, inappropriate timing of feeds, and use of supplementary and/or complement feeds and length of stay in hospital all influence the success of breast-feeding.

Breast-feeding

The most appropriate nutrition for an infant is the child's own mother's milk with very few exeptions even amongst sick infants. Full-term infants can suckle within minutes of birth and indeed it is recommended they should do so in order that successful breast-feeding is established. Exclusive breast-feeding in the first 6 months of life can provide full nutrition (Ahn & MacLean 1980, Rattigan *et al.* 1981) and together with weaning solids and a source of vitamins A, D, C is recommended until 8 to 10 months when the child has been weaned onto a cup and solids. Breast-feeding can continue even into the second year of life, and has advantages particularly where there is a family history of atopia and food allergic disease (Saarinen *et al.* 1979; Soothill 1982).

Successful breast-feeding depends on the establishment of the correct technique, unlimited suckling time and unlimited number of feeds. The mother needs to be tuned to her baby's needs.

COLOSTRUM

Colostrum is produced by the mammary glands for the first few days after birth and varies in composition. It is particularly rich in protein containing up to 9 times that of mature human milk. Approximately one fifth of the protein is casein and the remainder is soluble whey protein of which about half is secretory IgA (McClelland *et al.* 1978). The protein has a specific amino acid composition rich in tryptophan needed for regulating nitrogen synthesis, and arginine which stimulates the urea cycle. It is also rich in antibodies, cells, minerals and vitamins A, D and B_{12} with less fat than mature human milk. The composition of colostrum is given in Table 1.4. An anti-trypsin factor in colostrum prevents the digestion of antibodies, and much of the protein is therefore not absorbed.

Frequent suckling by the infant in the first few days not only increases the quantity of colostrum consumed but stimulates the breast to produce milk and establish breast-feeding. After birth, first colostrum and then milk satisfies the nutritional needs of the infant. Glucose water (or water) is unnecessary except when neonatal hypoglycaemia is present, and this is best prevented by early feeding, from the first few minutes of life.

MATURE HUMAN MILK

The transition from colostrum to mature milk is gradual. The composition of human milk is given in Tables 1.5 to 1.6. It provides

Table 1.4 Composition of human colostrum.

Substance	Unit	Amount/100 ml colostrum
Total protein	g	10.0^a, 1.4 to 2.3^d
Energy	kJ	226 to 306^d
	kcal	54 to 73^d
Fat	g	2.9^b, 1.9 to 3^d
Lactose	g	5.3 to 6.3^{bd}
Minerals		
Sodium	mmol	2.1 to 4.2^{bd}
Potassium	mmol	1.5 to 1.9^{bd}
Calcium	mmol	0.8^b, 0.6 to 1.2^d
Magnesium	mmol	0.16^b, 0.13 to 1.8^d
Phosphorus	mmol	0.5^{bd}
Vitamins		
Vitamin A	μg	126.0^b
Vitamin D (water soluble)	μg	1.78^c
Vitamin C	mg	4.4^b to 7.2^d
Thiamin	μg	15.0^b to 19.0^{bd}
Riboflavin	μg	30.0^{bd}
Nicotinic acid	μg	75.0^{bd}
Vitamin B_{12}	μg	0.045^b to 0.063^{bd}
Pantothenic acid	μg	183.0^{bd}
Biotin	μg	0.1^b

Sources
[a] McClelland *et al.* 1978 ⎫ Composition on 2nd day,
[b] Macy & Kelly 1961 ⎬ post partum
[c] Lakdawala & Widdowson 1977 ⎭
[d] Lentner 1981. Composition during first five days post partum

the infant's nutritional requirement provided adequate lactation is established. Demand feeding is essential and to increase supply, more frequent feeds should be given for a few days to allow suckling to stimulate milk production. It has been suggested that the infant can in some way regulate energy intake to his or her own needs if allowed to demand feed (Ounsted & Sleigh 1975). Demand feeding in maternity units is recommended (DHSS 1983, revised) and was more common in the survey from 1980 than in 1975 (Martin & Monk 1982).

Satisfactory growth and development after birth is more certain when an infant is fed an adequate quantity of human milk. Breast-feeding failure does occur but this is commonly due to inappropriate advice and lack of practical help. An inadequate supply of breast milk is the commonest reason given for cessation of breast-feeding or the introduction of other foods, either complement feeds or solids (Martin & Monk 1982). Whitehead *et al.* (1980) and others have suggested milk production is inadequate to meet the increasing nutritional needs of the infant from about 3 months. However, others (Ahn & MacLean 1980; Rattigan *et al.* 1981; Chandra 1981) have reported higher and rising milk production beyond 3 months and Rattigan *et al.* (1981) in Australia showed that most of the women could satisfy dietary requirements of their infants by breast-feeding alone for 6 to 9 months, and some could do so for 12 months or more. By and large the mothers of bigger, faster growing babies produce more milk to meet their babies' needs than mothers of smaller babies and a number of women successfully breast-fed twins. Sub-optimal lactation performance, rather than an inability to produce milk, is the cause of breast-feeding failure, due to inappropriate technique, lack of stimulation by suckling, timed feeds, premature introduction of other foods or feeds and social factors including the mother's return to work both in the home as well as her 'professional' commitments. A 'doula', who provides maternal support (as seen in many third world countries) marvellously enhances a mother's self-confidence which is so crucial to breast-feeding success. A number of lay groups, for example, the National Childbirth Trust (NCT) Breast-feeding Promotion Group, LaLeche League, and Breast-feeding Mothers Association, together with the initial support of midwife and then health visitor can provide excellent sympathetic help and support in this country.

Recognition of breast-feeding failure as a cause of failure to thrive is important (Davies 1979). Some infants are fretful, others over-contented and are therefore more easily overlooked. Regular weighing of the infant, charted on growth percentile charts, should alert professionals and parents to the problem. Investigation of breast-feeding technique with practical advice on increasing lactation, e.g., an extra 2 breast feeds per day or if this is impractical introduction of suitable foods or feeds should be given as appropriate. The maternal diet should be adequate and the mother requires sufficient rest, even if obtained at unusual times, in order to maintain adequate lactation. Test weighing of the infant before and after each breast feed throughout 24 hours is more likely to suppress lactation than achieve better nutrition; a single test feed gives a false idea of the intake due to the natural variation between different feeds.

Many advantages of breast-feeding have been given and are well documented in *Artificial Feeds for the Young Infant* (DHSS 1980a), *Present Day Practice in Infant Feeding* (DHSS 1983, revised) and *The Collection and Storage of Human Milk* (DHSS 1981a).

Breast-feeding should be encouraged. It is best for baby nutritionally, has positive protection against infections and probably allergy, helps bonding between mother and child and is cheaper than artificial feeding, both for the mother once she is at home and for hospitals. Breast-fed infants get less infections than artificially fed infants, as breast milk contains antigens and other immune factors that prevent bacterial and virus infections (Narayanan *et al.* 1982a,b; Holmes *et al.* 1983).

The bioavailability of nutrients from human milk is optimal, for example, zinc is present in a complex ligand with protein which enhances its absorption, and iron is better absorbed.

Protein Quality and Quantity for Young Infants
The relatively low protein, high energy content of human milk (8%

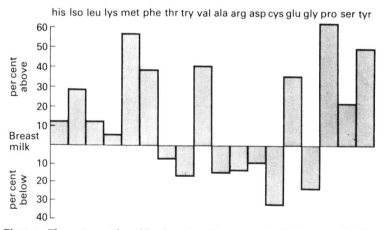

Fig. 1.1 The amino acid profile of cow's milk compared with human milk. (From FAO/WHO 1970. Reproduced with permission from the Food and Agriculture Organisation of the United Nations.)

energy from protein) is both easily digested and assimilated for growth. Human milk protein is low in casein and rich in lactalbumin compared to cow's milk. The amino acid composition of human milk protein is biologically most suited for growth in human infants. Cow's milk is over-rich in protein for the human infant and the proportion of amino acids is completely different to that of human milk (Fig.1.1) (Jelliffe & Jelliffe 1978).

Cow's milk protein is low in cystine, arginine, tryptophan, and taurine; all of these are essential amino acids in the newborn, e.g., as cystathionase enzyme activity to convert methionine to cystine is immature at birth, human milk ensures adequate cystine intake for taurine production; both cystine and taurine are essential for brain growth. Taurine is also important for bile salt metabolism and therefore fat absorption. Milks with a whey:casein ratio of 60:40 partially correct the imbalance of amino acids except possibly for tryptophan; they are recommended for all infants and especially for those of low birth weight or born prematurely, as the source of protein if human milk is not used. Some formulae are fortified with taurine. Casein-based formulae are poorly absorbed unless predigested by hydrolysation and need amino acid supplementation of cystine, tryptophan and possibly tyrosine if used for neonates.

After absorption amino acids reach the liver where they are used for protein synthesis and other anabolic processes. Amino acids in excess of anabolic needs are degraded for adenosine triphosphate (ATP) production, gluconeogenesis or liponeogenesis and the amino groups converted to ammonia for conversion into urea (Smith & Francis 1982). Neonatal immaturity of the liver enzymes for amino acid degradation can give rise to elevated blood amino acids. This is most likely to occur in preterm infants, in the presence of high protein intakes, imbalance of amino acids, in low birth weight infants or any situation which increases gluconeogenesis such as under-nutrition, infection or other causes of catabolism. Most commonly the raised blood amino acids are phenylalanine, tyrosine and/or methionine (Smith & Francis 1982) and these raised levels may persist for several months (Snyderman *et al.* 1968). The clinical significance of these transient amino acid elevations remain in doubt. However transient tyrosinaemia may cause intellectual deficits which only become apparent in later childhood (Menkes *et al.* 1972; Mamunes *et. al.* 1976). Also a follow-up study of low birth weight infants given 4% casein feeds had a lower IQ at 7 years old than those fed feeds containing 2% casein (Goldman *et al.* 1974).

It is now recommended that young infants should not be given feeds containing more than 2 g protein per 100 ml (DHSS 1980a) or protein intakes of more than 4 g protein/kg actual weight per day.

Fat

Human milk contains lipase and hence human milk fat is particularly well absorbed. It is relatively high in essential unsaturated fatty acids. The fat content of human milk increases during the feed, the hind milk having a higher energy and fat content. It is therefore important that the infant actually gets this milk by appropriate milking of the breast during suckling.

Changes in the fat composition occur gradually throughout lactation and could be physiologically significant to the neonate (Crawford et al. 1976). Fat is an important component of the brain and the nervous system. Early in lactation human milk phosphoglycerides are rich in long chain polyunsaturated fatty acids with a gradual change to long chain monosaturated fatty acids which together with cholesterol facilitate myelination of the brain. The latter starts before birth and continues until about 4 years of age (Dobbing & Sands 1973). The newborn however is capable of synthesizing these fatty acids from their precursors linoleic and linolenic acid.

Iron

Iron status in the newborn depends on the iron content of the body at birth, growth and the balance between losses and intake. Healthy full-term breast-fed infants can maintain satisfactory iron status in the first months of life (McMillan et al. 1976) due to the efficiency of iron absorption and utilization from human milk. The amount of iron in human milk therefore appears to be adequate as the sole source of exogenous iron (DHSS 1980a). Iron is poorly absorbed by infants from formula milk and microcytic anaemia and occult gastrointestinal bleeding with iron loss have been reported (DHSS 1980a).

The availability of iron from foods and fortified milks is uncertain and supersaturates the human milk lactoferrin rendering it inactive in inhibiting bacterial growth. There is some suggestion that other sources of iron interfere with the availability of iron from human milk thus reducing rather than improving iron status. Iron absorption increases with increasing need (Van Campen 1974). The nutritional anaemias of newborns is documented by Haworth & Evans (1981).

Vitamins

Vitamin D sulphate has been found in the aqueous fraction of human milk (Sahashi *et al.* 1967; Lakdawala & Widdowson 1977). This together with the small amount of fat-soluble vitamin D provides 1 µg vitamin D per 100 ml which is a similar quantity of vitamin D to that in fortified milks. Providing vitamin D sulphate is biologically active, together with the clinical observation that breast-fed infants rarely get rickets, it is probably unnecessary to supplement vitamin D in fully breast-fed infants, providing the mother's diet is adequate.

Maternal Diet

An integral part of infant nutrition and breast-feeding success is the mother's nutritional intake, provision of adequate fluid to meet her thirst, together with adequate rest. The lactating mother needs approximately 1700 to 2500 kJ (400 to 600 kcal) extra per day compared to other women. This extra energy should be provided as a range of foods and snacks such as wholemeal bread, sandwiches and drinks like tea, coffee, fruit juice and of course, free access to water. These items should also be available at night, as 2 to 4 breast feeds are usually given between the mother's evening meal and breakfast, the following day.

Milk intake in the maternal diet is not essential for successful breast-feeding, but for the majority ½ to 1 pint of milk per day is ideal and supplies important calcium, riboflavin and protein. Many women complain of hunger and then gorge inappropriately on fruit or chocolate. Excess of any food may allow sensitizing of the baby through the unchanged protein which transfers from her diet to the milk. In a few instances, such sensitizing can later trigger off food allergies such as eczema, and the mother may need to exclude the causative food from her diet in order to control symptoms in the infant. The maternal diet should normally contain generous quantities of wholegrain cereals, fruit, vegetables and wholemeal bread. These also help to alleviate constipation which can be a problem. A wide variety of food should be included. Protein should be supplied by meat, egg, cheese, fish, pulses, cereals and nuts. Breast-feeding has the additional advantage of using maternal energy stores, thus helping the woman to ultimately return to her normal former weight.

Artificial feeds

The development of sophisticated artificial feeds has undoubtedly made bottle-feeding safer than formerly, but no artificial feed can completely mimic the nutritional and protective properties of human milk. Artificial feeds are only as good as modern technology and economics permit. The marketing practice of milk manufacturers should be monitored to ensure their methods comply with the *International Code of Marketing of Breast Milk Substitutes* (WHO 1981). The code aims to prevent mothers being unduly persuaded either directly or indirectly to bottle-feed.

Recommended International Standards for Foods for Infants and Children. Joint FAO/WHO Food Standards Programme. Codex Alimentarius Commission (FAO/WHO 1976) and in the UK *Artificial Feeds for the Young Infant* (DHSS 1980a) provide guidelines (Table 1.5) to ensure nutritionally adequate safe alternatives to breast-feeding are available. As yet no exact guidelines for trace nutrients are given due to insufficient knowledge.

All non-breast-fed young infants should be fed a modified milk which meets these guidelines. A number of such milks are available (Table 1.6a and b). Ethnic groups with religious food laws should be directed to the appropriate formulae e.g., SMA (J. Wyeth) contains oleo oil (beef fat) which is unacceptable to vegetarian, Moslem and Jewish families; vegans will require an appropriate soya-modified formulae e.g., S Formula (Cow & Gate) if the infant is not breast-fed. These milks should be used until at least 6 months of age and there are nutritional advantages in their use in bottle-fed infants until 8 to 10 months when the child can have milk from a cup and is having a wide range of weaning solids. Cow's milk, 'filled' milks in which butterfat is replaced with alternative fats, evaporated milk, partially skimmed, skimmed milk and goat's milk are all unsuitable, as they do not meet the nutritional needs of the young infant whose immature kidneys and liver enzymes system cannot handle the high solute and protein content of these milks. 'Follow-on' milks, e.g., Progress (J. Wyeth) can be introduced as an alternative to cow's milk from 6 months of age onwards in conjunction with appropriate solids.

Infants should be demand-fed whether by bottle or breast. The formula should be aseptically prepared, correctly diluted and in the early months of life approximately 150 to 200 ml/kg weight per day should be offered on demand in 4 to 8 feeds per day, traditionally at about 3- to 4-hourly intervals.

A quick method of calculating feed volume to offer on demand is: For 200 ml/kg per day give 25 ml × weight in kg × approx. 3-hourly
× 8 feeds

For 150 ml/kg per day give 30 ml × weight in kg × approx. 4-hourly
× 5 feeds

The individual infant will deviate from this plan but this guide
ensures the infant is offered adequate for his or her fluid and
nutritional needs. Force-feeding should be avoided and the child's
growth and contentment used as a monitor as with breast-fed infants.

Of the modified milks available, the whey-based milks more
closely mimic the human milk amino acid and fatty acid profiles, as
they contain a higher % whey protein and a mixture of vegetable
plus animal fat or butterfat. There are no significant differences
between brands of these formulae. Some are now supplemented
with taurine. The milks are available as 'ready-to-feed' formulae,
powdered milk and some as liquid concentrate. The latter due to
the heat treatment used during manufacture are lower in
sensitizing capacity or allergenicity than 'ready-to-feed', and these
latter are less sensitizing than formulae made from powdered milks
when tested in the guinea pig model (McLaughlin *et al.* 1981). All
of the modified milk formulae are less sensitizing than 'doorstep'
cow's milk. This is important in patients at risk of atopia and food
allergic disease, and temporarily after gastroenteritis and infection
when there is an increased risk of sensitizing. However, highly
heat-treated milks contain lactulose formed during processing and
storage of liquid milk. It can precipitate diarrhoea or loose stools
and changes in gut flora have been reported (Adachi & Patton 1961;
Mendez & Olano 1979). The availability of the amino acid lysine is
reduced by heating due to the malliard reaction, and vitamin losses
also occur, though the latter are made good by the manufacturer
adding supplements.

Cow's milk and goat's milk are not recommended for infants
under 6 months (DHSS 1980a, 1983, revised). Simple dilution will
not produce a feed of optimal nutritional content. However, a
temporary feed can be devised for use when a modified milk is not
available. The recipe given in Table 1.7 is adapted from Cameron &
Hofvander (1983).

Breast-feeding, although it does not always prevent the
development of allergy, is the most satisfactory means of avoiding
food allergy (Matthew *et al.* 1977; Saarinen *et al.* 1979; Soothill
1982). It is recommended as the sole source of nutrition for at least
the first 4 months and preferably 6 months in those infants at
greatest risk, such as those whose parents have a history of atopic
disease (DHSS 1983, revised). Opinions differ but soya milk is
probably the most practical alternative if breast-feeding is not

Table 1.5 Composition of mature human milk and nutritional guidelines for the composition of artificial feeds per 100 ml. (From DHSS 1983, revised.)

		Mean values for pooled samples of mature human milk[a,b]	Guidelines for artificial feeds[b]	
			Minimum	Maximum
Energy	kJ	293	270	315
	kcal	70	65	75
Protein	g	1.3[c]	1.5[c]	2[c]
	g		1.2[d]	2[d]
Lactose	g	7	2.5	8
Total carbohydrate	g		4.8	10
Fat	g	4.2	2.3	5
Vitamins				
A	μg	60	40	150
D	μg	0.01	0.7	1.3
E[e]	mg	0.35	0.3	
K	μg	0.21[f]	1.5	
Thiamin	μg	16	13	
Riboflavin	μg	30	30	
Nicotinic acid	μg	230	230	
B_6	μg	6	5	N/S
B_{12}	μg	0.01	0.01	
Total folate	μg	5.2	3	
Pantothenic acid	μg	260	200	
Biotin	μg	0.76	0.5	
C	mg	3.8	3	
Minerals				
Sodium	mmol	0.7	0.7	1.5
Potassium	mmol	1.5	1.3	2.6
Chloride	mmol	1.2	1.1	2.3
Calcium[g]	mmol	0.9	0.8	3
Phosphorus	mmol	0.5	0.5	1.9
Magnesium	mmol	0.12	0.12	0.49
Iron[h]	μmol	1.36	1.25	12.5
Copper	μmol	0.6		
Zinc	μmol	4.5	N/S[h]	N/S[h]
Iodine	μmol	0.06		

[a] DHSS 1977.

[b] DHSS 1980a.

[c] Cow's milk protein in which casein to whey ratio is unadjusted (type a milks, i.e. modified milks).

[d] Casein whey ratio is similar to that of human milk (type b milks, i.e. whey-based milks).

[e] The ratio of tocopherol (mg) to polyunsaturated fatty acids (g) should be not less than 0.4:1.02.

[f] Haroon *et al.* 1982.

[g] The ratio of calcium to phosphorus should not be less than 1.2:1.0 or more than 2.2:1.0.

[h] Guidelines for trace elements other than iron are not set.

Chapter 1

Table 1.6 Composition of various infant feeds per 100 ml. (Data supplied by manufacturers 1984).

Product[a] (Company)	% Solution	Protein[b] Tot. g	L %	C %	Carbohydrate Tot. g	Type	Fat[c] Tot. g	Sat. %	Unsat. %	Energy kJ/kcal	Osmolality mmol/kg	Renal solute mmol/100 ml[d]	Minerals Na+ mmol	K+ mmol	Ca++ mmol	P- mmol	Mg- mmol	Fe+ µmol	Cu+ µmol	Zn+ µmol	Cl- mmol
Human milk (Mature)	Liquid	1.3	60.0[e]	40.0[e]	7.2	Lactose[e]	4.1	50.1	47.4	289/69	264	8.4	0.6	1.5	0.9	0.5	0.1	1.3	0.6	4.3	1.2
Human milk (Transitional)	Liquid	2.0	60.0	40.0	6.9	Lactose	3.7	50.1	47.4	281/67	—	14.2	2.1	1.7	0.6	0.5	0.1	1.3	0.6	—	2.4
1 Whey-based modified milks (Ready-to-feed or reconstituted powder)																					
Aptamil[f] (Milupa)	14.0	1.5	60.0	40.0	7.2	Lactose	3.6	51.8	48.2	273/65	305/l	14.0	0.8	—	1.4	1.1	—	12.5	0.4	4.6	—
Gold Cup SMA [S26][f] (J. Wyeth)	13.0	1.5	60.0	40.0	7.2	Lactose	3.6	46.7	53.1 (Soyalecithin, veg. & beef fat)	274/65	300	9.1	0.7	1.4	1.1	1.1	0.2	12.0	0.8	7.6	1.2
Nan (Nestlé)	13.0	1.6	60.0	40.0	7.3	Lactose	3.4	46.0	48.0	276/66	—	10.6	0.8	1.9	1.1	1.0	0.2	14.3	0.6	7.6	1.5
Premium (Cow & Gate)	12.5	1.5	60.0	40.0	7.3	Lactose	3.6	41.1	56.2 (Veg. & butter fat)	275/66	290	9.6	0.8	1.7	1.4	0.9	0.2	8.9	0.6	6.1	1.3
Osterfeed (Farley)	13.0	1.45	61.4	38.6	7.0	Lactose	3.8	38.7	61.3 (Veg. & butter fat, soyalecithin)	284/68	300	9.4	0.8	1.5	0.9	1.0	0.2	11.6	0.7	5.4	1.3
2 Modified milks (non-whey-based) (Ready-to-feed or reconstituted powder)																					
White Cap SMA[f] (J. Wyeth)	13.0	1.5	20.0	80.0	7.2	Lactose	3.6	46.7	53.1 (Veg. & beef fat)	275/65	295	10.3	0.9	1.9	1.4	1.4	0.2	12.0	0.8	7.6	1.3
Ostermilk Complete Formula (Farley)	13.9	1.7	23.0	77.0	8.6	Lactose Maltodextrin	2.6	—	— (Veg. & butter fat)	273/65	210	11.5	1.4	1.8	1.5	1.6	0.3	11.6	0.6	5.0	1.6
Ostermilk 2 (Farley)	13.5	1.8	23.0	77.0	8.3	Lactose Maltodextrin	2.4	60.0	40.0 (Butter fat & veg. oils)	260/62	270	12.2	1.3	2.0	1.6	1.7	0.3	11.6	0.3	3.4	1.7
Babymilk Plus (Cow & Gate)	12.5	1.9	20.0	80.0	7.3	Lactose	3.4	41.1	56.2 (Veg. & butter fat)	275/66	310	13.0	1.1	2.6	2.1	1.8	0.3	8.9	0.6	6.4	1.7
Milumil[f] (Milupa)	14.0	1.9	20.0	80.0	8.4	Lactose Maltodextrin Amylose	3.1	53.7	46.3	286/68	360/l	12.5	1.2	2.2	1.8	1.8	0.3	12.5	0.2	3.4	1.3

3 Preterm low birth weight formulae (Ready-to-feed only)

Product	Form	Protein (g)	L[b]	C[b]	CHO (g)	CHO source	Fat (g)	Sat[c]	Unsat[c]	(fat type)	kJ/kcal										
Nenatal (Cow & Gate)	Liquid	1.8	61.1	38.9	7.4	Lactose Glucose Maltodextrin	4.5	47.9	52.1	(Corn oil & MCT)	318/76	340	10.7	0.9	1.5	2.5	1.6	0.6	14.3	1.2	12.3	1.1
Prematalac (Cow & Gate)	Liquid	2.4	60.0	40.0	6.6	Lactose	5.0	51.4	48.6	(Butter fat & veg. oils)	330/79	342/l	16.9	2.6	2.4	1.7	1.7	0.5	11.6	0.8	6.1	2.3
Gold Cap SMA / Low Birth Weight SMA[f] (J. Wyeth)	Liquid	2.0	60.0	40.0	8.6	Lactose Maltodextrin	4.4	48.9	50.9	(Veg., oleo & MCT oils)	335/80	268	12.8	1.4	1.9	1.9	1.3	0.3	12	1.1	7.6	1.5
Preamptamil[f] (Milupa)	Liquid	2.1	48.0	52.0	8.3	Lactose	3.6	46.9	53.1	(Veg. & butter fat)	308/74	350	13.2	1.5	2.1	1.5	1.5	0.3	12.5	1.6	15.4	1.3
Osterprem (Farley)	Liquid	2.0	39.5	60.5	7.0	Lactose Maltodextrin	4.9	39.5	60.5	(Veg. & butter fat)	334/80	300	13.3	2.1	1.5	1.8	1.1	0.2	0.7	1.9	15.3	1.7

4 Milks for infants over 6 months

Product	Form	Protein (g)	L[b]	C[b]	CHO (g)	CHO source	Fat (g)	Sat[c]	Unsat[c]	(fat type)	kJ/kcal										
Cow's milk	Liquid	3.3	18.0	82.0	4.7	Lactose	3.8	61.1	34.8		272/65	—	22.0	2.2	3.9	3.0	3.1	0.5	0.9	0.3	5.4	2.7
Goat's milk	Liquid	3.3	—	—	4.6	Lactose	4.5	—	—		296/71	—	23.2	1.7	4.6	3.3	3.5	0.8	0.7	0.8	4.6	3.7
Progress 'Follow on' Formula (J. Wyeth)	—	2.9	60.0	40.0	8.0	Lactose Maltodextrin	2.6	44.6	55.4		272/65	—	18.2	1.7	2.7	2.9	3.0	0.4	14.3	0.9	6.6	2.1

5 Modified soya milks

Product	Form	Protein (g)	L[b]	C[b]	CHO (g)	CHO source	Fat (g)	Sat[c]	Unsat[c]	(fat type)	kJ/kcal										
S Formula[a] (Cow & Gate)	12.7	1.8	(Soy Isolate & l-Methionine)		6.7	Glucose syrup	3.6			(Vegetable oils)	280/67	165	10.8	0.8	1.7	1.4	0.9	0.2	8.9	0.6	6.2[h]	1.1
Prosobee[f] (Mead Johnson)	13.0	2.0	(Soy Isolate & l-Methionine)		6.7	Corn syrup solids	3.6			(Coconut & corn oil)	281/67	160	11.7	1.1	1.5	1.5	1.3	0.3	21.5	0.9	7.6[h]	1.1
Wysoy[f] (J. Wyeth)	13.5	2.1	(Soy Isolate & l-Methionine)		6.9	Sucrose + corn syrup solids	3.6			(Oleic, beef fat, corn & coconut oils)	280/67	242	12.2	0.9	1.9	1.6	1.4	0.3	12.1	0.8	5.7[h]	1.0

6 Hydrolyzed protein formulae

Product	Form	Protein (g)	L[b]	C[b]	CHO (g)	CHO source	Fat (g)	Sat[c]	Unsat[c]	(fat type)	kJ/kcal										
Pregestimil (Mead Johnson)	15.0	1.9	(Hydrolyzed casein & cystine tyrosine, tryptophan)		9.1	Corn syrup solids + tapioca starch	2.7			(Corn oil, MCT & soyalecithin)	287/68	338	12.5	1.4	1.9	1.6	1.4	0.3	23.0	0.9	6.0	1.6
Nutramigen[i] (Mead Johnson)	15.0	2.3	(Hydrolyzed casein)		8.9	Sucrose + tapioca starch	2.7			(Corn oil)	290/69	443	13.8	1.4	1.8	1.6	1.6	0.3	23.0	1.0	6.6	1.4

a All contain a range of vitamins with the exception of cow's and goat's milks. However children's Vitamin A, D, C, Drops supplement is recommended except with Osterprem (Farley) from 1 month till at least 2 years and preferably 5 years old.

b L = Lactalbumin and whey as % total protein. C = Casein as % total protein. (Type of protein in parentheses.)

c Sat. = saturated fat as % total fat. Unsat. = mono- and polyunsaturated fats as % total fat. (Type of fat in parentheses.)

d Renal solute load is the sum of (protein × 4) + mmol Na^+ + mmol K^+ + mmol Cl^- per 100 ml.

e Foman 1984.

f Also available as liquid concentrate.

g May 1984 reformulation.

h Zinc phytate molar ration 1:9.

i Not recommended for infants under 3 months.

Table 1.7 Simple modification of milk(s) for a temporary infant feed. (Adapted from Cameron & Hofvander 1983.)

---

125 ml boiled cow's milk or boiled goat's milk or 25 ml unsweetened evaporated milk

15 g sugar or lactose or 20 g honey

Boiled water to 200 ml

Each 100 ml contains approximately 292 kJ (70 kcal) and 2 to 2.1 g protein. Children's Vitamin A, D, C, Drops (Welfare Food Supplies) are recommended and if goat's milk is used, folic acid and B_{12} supplements are advised.

possible (Glaser & Johnstone 1953), though the casein hydrolysate formulae are least likely to cause sensitization but are expensive (*Drugs & Therapeutics Bulletin* Editorial, 1983). A suitable, modified soya formula (Table 1.6) should be selected (DHSS 1983, revised) such as 'S' Formula, Prosobee (Mead Johnson) or Wysoy (J. Wyeth). Delayed introduction of solids, particularly the high risk allergens such as cow's milk, egg, nuts, citrus fruit, berry fruit and wheat may delay or decrease the incidence of some forms of food allergic disease such as eczema (Fergusson *et al.* 1981).

FEED PREPARATION

Correct reconstitution of infant feeds in essential. The standard dilution for powdered modified milks made in the UK is 1 level scoop of powder to each 30 ml (1 ounce) measured water, using the scoop supplied with the product. In hospitals more accurate reconstitution is achieved by weighing the powder and making standard solutions of 12½ to 15% as recommended for the particular product. Over-concentration, particularly if inadequate water is available as a result of gastroenteritis or fever, due to the infant's immature kidney being unable to concentrate urine, can lead to hypernatraemia and dehydration. The latter can lead to brain damage and even death. Excess concentration and high osmolar feeds can lead to malabsorption with faecal losses. Long-term over-concentration can result in obesity. Over-dilute feeds lead to inadequate intake, failure to thrive, malnutrition with its subsequent risk of infection and further malnutrition.

Domestic drinking water is suitable for feed reconstitution but health authorities should ensure that it meets accepted standards of quality so that infants are not exposed to excess lead, nitrates or sodium which can be harmful (DHSS 1983, revised). Softened water and bottled waters with high sodium content are unsuitable.

The water recepticle should be freshly filled, boiled and then cooled, the water measured and then the measured scoops of powder added and dissolved.

Aseptic preparation of feeds is essential to prevent infection. Sterilized or disinfected bottles, teats, teat caps and feed making equipment are essential (Wharton & Berger 1976) for all bottle feeds whatever the age of the child. Sterilizing tablets (hypochlorite) are available for home use.

In hospitals, a centralized milk formula room is optimal, using autoclaved bottles and equipment, aseptic feed reconstitution and bottling by trained staff 7 days a week. Terminal pasteurization of feeds is recommended such as 67.5°C for 4 minutes, which we use, 63°C for 30 minutes or equivalent; the feeds should be quickly cooled, then refrigerated for up to 24 hours until required for use. Pasteurization is preferable to sterilization which destroys nutrients due to the malliard reaction, caramelizes sugar(s) and forms lactulose and destroys vitamins. Ideally, feeds should not be heated above 70°C. 'Ready-to-feed' formulae reduce the number of feeds requiring such preparation and hence equipment and staffing, but not necessarily space as they are bulky to store. The high cost of 'ready-to-feed' may largely offset the modified milk powder, equipment and staffing costs of a centralized milk room, but both are more expensive than breast-feeding even for the mother at home as well as in hospitals. In the UK at present 'ready-to-feed' is only available for hospitals and institutions.

Preparation of a whole day's feeds is only advised when a refrigerator is available for storing, otherwise feeds should be made immediately before use. Refrigerated feeds can be warmed over hot (not boiling) water or fed cold (Blumenthal *et al.* 1980) except to sick or low birth weight infants. Bottle warmers, thermos flasks and polystyrene containers which keep made-up feeds warm should not be used, as microbial contamination can quickly multiply to inappropriately high levels.

Cool boiled water or, after the first 6 weeks, dilute (natural) fruit juice should be offered to bottle-fed infants if they are thirsty or cry between feeds, during hot weather, or if the baby has a temperature, diarrhoea or vomiting. Fruit juices are preferably given from a spoon or cup and should be discouraged at night. Sugar, sugar drinks and dummies or 'dinky feeders' increase the incidence of dental caries and should normally be avoided. Breast-fed infants do not require additional water even in hot weather, though extra breast feeds can be offered when desired.

Expressed Breast Milk

The mother whose infant initially cannot suckle may supply her own milk for the baby. The mother expresses her milk (EBM) into sterile bottles supplied for the purpose. The EBM is refrigerated or frozen until it is required for the infant. Breast pumps are frequently used to express the milk and are either the hand type e.g., Kaneson (Yanase Waitch K. K, Japan, distributed in the UK by Kimal Scientific Products Ltd., Uxbridge) or various electric models, e.g., Egnell (Ameda Ltd.). A number of new brands are currently being evaluated. Breast pumps require careful sterilization and/or disinfection of all parts that come into contact with the milk to reduce the risk of microbial contamination. Bacteriological monitoring is essential to ensure adequate standards are maintained. However pasteurization is unnecessary and destroys some of the protective factors of the milk.

HUMAN MILK BANKS

Some women donate human milk to milk banks for those infants whose own mother cannot supply enough for the baby's needs. Donated milk may be 'drip' breast milk, collected in sterilized breast nipple shields then decanted into sterile bottles, or expressed by the woman for the milk bank while continuing to breast-feed her own infant. The donated milk is frozen to store it and is bacteriologically monitored and/or pasteurized to ensure its safety (DHSS 1981a). Special human milk pasteurizers, e.g., made

Table 1.8 Average composition of human pooled expressed and drip human milks. (From DHSS 1981.)

		Expressed milk[a]	Drip milk[b]
Energy	kcal/l	700	480
	kJ/l	2900	2000
Protein	g/l	10.7	10
Lactose	g/l	74	65
Fat	g/l	42	22
Sodium	mmol/l	6.4	5.5
Potassium	mmol/l	15	16.1
Calcium	mmol/l	8.7	6.9
Magnesium	mmol/l	1.2	1.2

[a] DHSS 1977.

[b] Gibbs *et al.* 1977.

by Vickers, Colgate can be used to keep the maximum protective immunological factors in the milk. Guidelines on the *Collection and Storage of Human Milk* (DHSS 1981a) outline the dilemma surrounding the use of pasteurized *versus* unpasteurized human milk for sick infants. The handling, collection, storage and feeding of human milk requires special attention to detail to ensure the important protective factors are not lost, but the milk is microbially safe.

Nutritional factors must not be overlooked. 'Drip' milk is of a lower energy and fat content then EBM (DHSS 1981a) (Table 1.8) and may require fortification with an appropriate energy source. Supplements of

1 to 3 g glucose polymer carbohydrate
and/or 2 g fat e.g., 4 ml Prosparol (Duncan Flockhart Ltd.),
Calogen (SHS) or Liquigen (SHS)
to each 100 ml 'drip' breast milk

can be used to restore the energy deficit. Many milk banks use a mixture of expressed and 'drip' milk. A quick method for determining the fat content of the banked human milk has been suggested by Lucas *et al.* (1978) so that the energy content can be supplemented appropriately.

There are also possibilities for modifying human milk by the addition of concentrates of some of its own constituents such as fat and protein (Lucas *et al.* 1980; Williams & Baum 1984), to make a more appropriate composition to meet the nutritional needs of the low birth weight infant. If human milk concentrates are not available a supplement of 5 g Pregestimil (Mead Johnson) to 100 ml human milk provides a fortified formula which has been occasionally used for infants with increased nutritional requirements such as those of low birth weight or with cystic fibrosis.

LOW BIRTH WEIGHT INFANTS

Percentile charts relating fetal measurement to gestational age are available (Tanner & Thomson 1970). Low birth weight infants grow and develop less well than normal infants (Neligan *et al.* 1976). Such infants are prone to hypoglycaemia and need carbohydrate and energy as a matter of urgency as energy reserves are very limited (see Table 1.15). They should be fed immediately after birth. Davies & Russell (1968) showed a reduced incidence of hypoglycaemia and hyperbilirubinaemia in these infants and improved mental and neurological status later in childhood when they were fed liberal amounts of undiluted breast milk from immediately after birth. The brain's metabolism uses at least 65% of basal (fasting) metabolic energy in the young infant and brain growth is rapid immediately before and after birth and should be interrupted for as short a time as possible (Dobbing 1974).

Infants who are born before 34 weeks gestation or with birth weights of less than 1.5 kg have increased nutritional requirements, are more prone to enzyme immaturity and the infant may be unable to suck and swallow adequately. Nasogastric or nasojejunal feeding or parenteral nutrition are required.

The survival of these very low birth weight infants means neonatal nutrition has become increasingly important. The optimal rate of growth for these infants is not known (Burman 1982; DHSS 1981a) and there is no agreement on either the nutritional requirements or best type of feeding (DHSS 1981a; Brooke et al. 1982; Eyal et al. 1982; Lucas et al. 1984).

Atkinson et al. (1978, 1980) have shown that the milk of mothers of preterm infants during the first month of lactation is higher in nitrogen and macro-minerals than the milk from mothers who have had full-term infants. Better growth and improved nutritional balances were found when infants were fed their own mother's milk (Atkinson et al. 1980). The higher nitrogen content of preterm milk was observed by Brooke et al. (1982) but nitrogen absorption was reported as no better than in infants fed other milks. Other reasons for the use of human milk in these infants include the anti-infective and immunological properties (Narayanan 1982a) and its biologically available nutrients. Relatively poor growth however has been reported in low birth weight infants fed pooled human milk (Davies 1977). This may be partially related to the lower energy value of 'drip' milk (Table 1.8) (DHSS 1981a) and technique of feeding which can markedly reduce the quantity of fat ingestion (Narayanan et al. 1984) and therefore energy intake of the baby. Pasteurization destroys lipase (Williams & Baum 1984) and therefore reduces fat availability (Williamson et al. 1978a,b); freezing alters fat globule size and increases the adhesion of fat to the sides of the storage receptacle (DHSS 1981a) and feeding equipment.

Frequently very ill and preterm infants cannot suck or swallow and require tube feeding by fine bore nasogastric tube instead of a bottle. The volumes must be measured accurately by syringe for bolus feeds or syringe pump for continuous feeds, as even small volume differences may be critical. Adult tube feed equipment is unsuitable. Great care to identify enteral feeds given by nasogastric or nasojejunal tube is essential. Even the positioning of the syringe pump and length of tubing can affect the amount of fat and energy the baby receives. Hence bolus feeds are preferable if they are tolerated, but may need to be given hourly. The length of nasogastric tube should be as short as possible but compatible with ease of nursing. The syringe pump used for administering continuous enteral feeds should ideally be positioned at an angle with the nozzle uppermost but the syringe below the level of the infant (Narayanan *et al.* 1984) to ensure maximum fat intake from the feed is received by the infant.

Other nutritional deficiencies have been reported (Burman 1982; Lucas *et al.* 1984) including osteoporosis, rickets, trace mineral deficiencies and temporary sodium depletion in low birth weight infants.

Suggestions have been made regarding the role of human milk in the prevention of necrotizing enterocolitis (Barlow *et al.* 1974). This has recently been disputed, with growing evidence that enteral feeding is involved in the pathogenesis of this condition. Eyal *et al.* (1982) have shown a reduced incidence when enteral feeds (human milk or formulae) were delayed for 2 to 3 weeks in very low birth weight infants who are at greatest risk of necrotizing enterocolitis. Nutrition was supplied parenterally.

The nutritional needs of the low birth weight infant have been suggested by the American Academy of Pediatrics Committee on Nutrition (1977) and Ziegler *et al.* (1981) in their *Textbook of Nutritional Requirements of the Preterm Infant*. The multicentre low birth weight feeding project based at Cambridge (Lucas *et al.* 1984) has provided additional information on the special needs of this group. Particular attention should be paid to increased requirements but nutrients in excess of requirement for growth put a load on different homeostatic mechanisms of the body, especially on those related to renal and hepatic function. Too large a margin of safety may lead to adverse effects because of functional immaturity. Excess protein increases the risk of metabolic acidosis, hyperammonaemia and transient hyperaminoacidaemia or uraemia and dehydration due to excess renal solute load.

Optimal protein intakes for low birth weight infants have not been firmly established. A number of studies using different formulae are being reported and a variety of preterm and low birth weight formulae (Table 1.6,**3**) have recently become available. The differing intakes of nutrients can influence the outcome and a limiting amount of any essential nutrient will inhibit growth. Such factors must be borne in mind when interpreting the results of different studies, for example Lucas *et al*. (1984) found the greatest weight gains were obtained in the infants fed a preterm formula compared to those fed the lower energy content human milk. Brooke *et al*. (1982) compared energy nitrogen balances and growth with 3 different formulae and pasteurized expressed breast milk and reported that nutritional parameters measured and growth were best on a preterm low birth weight type of formulae. No amino acid or trace mineral data were reported. Raiha *et al*. (1976) suggested that most low birth weight infants will, if given sufficient energy, grow satisfactorily on formulae providing 2.25 to 5 g/kg per day of cow's milk protein. However, Rassin *et al*. (1977) demonstrated tyrosine levels were twice as high when low birth weight infants were fed isocaloric formulae containing 3 g protein per 100 ml (whey:casein ratio 60:40) compared to those fed human milk; 1.5 g protein per 100 ml (whey:casein ratio 60:40) gave only slightly elevated levels. Tyrosine levels were further elevated if the milk contained predominantly casein (whey:casein ratio 18:82). Phenylalanine levels mimicked those of tyrosine. Follow-up studies of children in whom high protein intakes cause transient tyrosinaemia showed reduced IQ (Menkes *et al*. 1972; Mamunes *et al*. 1976; Goldman *et al*. 1974). Cystine and taurine are essential for the fetus and neonate especially if premature (Pohlandt 1974; Gaull *et al*. 1977).

Breast milk or formulae used for low birth weight infants should in the light of present knowledge provide at least 2 and not more than 4 g protein/kg actual weight per day. Adequate energy intake is essential. Breast milk or formulae should provide between 2.3 and 3 g protein per 420 kJ (100 kcal) i.e., 9.2 to 12% energy should come from protein with an amino acid profile similar to human milk. Other nutrients also require attention, especially in very low birth weight infants due to increased needs or losses.

Fluid due to increased insensible losses may need to exceed 150 ml to a maximum of 200 ml/kg per day, but fluid overload is not well tolerated. Energy in the range of 630 to 540 kJ (150 to 130 kcal)/kg per day should be provided at least by the end of the second week.

Sodium intake should be higher than for normal infants to prevent hyponatraemia, but must be monitored carefully (Roy *et al*.

1976) as the higher requirement may not persist. The renal solute must not exceed the kidneys' ability to concentrate urine.

Calcium requirements are increased and are possibly in the region of 180 mg calcium/kg per day in the very low birth weight infant, with a calcium:phosphorus ratio of 2:1 (Day *et al.* 1975; Burman 1982). Osteoporosis may occur. Calcium metabolism is inter-related to elevated vitamin D and phosphorus requirements.

Iron, zinc and copper requirements are all greater than for full-term neonates of normal birth weight (Ashkenazi *et al.* 1973). However, the complexity of trace mineral bioavailability and supplementation must be remembered (Aggett & Davies 1983) (see also Chapter 3).

Vitamins. Because of the low volume of feed taken by low birth weight infants, ensuring adequate vitamin intake necessitates either supplements or use of a formula with a higher density to volume or vitamins, e.g., Osterprem (Farley). Folic acid, B_{12}, vitamins D and E are particularly important (American Academy of Pediatrics on Nutrition 1977; Lucas *et al.* 1984).

Carbohydrate is an important source of energy. Intestinal lactase activity is present in the fetus from about 23 weeks and is quickly induced in most babies after birth. Lactose is usually tolerated satisfactorily but the occasional infant will have clinical lactose intolerance requiring an alternative source of carbohydrate. Pregestimil is currently the only nutritionally suitable lactose and sucrose-free formula available in the UK that could be recommended for the low birth weight infant. New formulae (Pepdite range by SHS) are being developed but require further evaluation in normal neonates before they can be considered for low birth weight infants.

Fat is also an essential source of energy but attention must be paid to both its absorption and provision of essential fatty acids. The role of lipase in human milk in the absorption of fat is extremely important, but is destroyed during pasteurization. As bile salt synthesis is limited in low birth weight infants poor fat absorption is common, especially from formulae. Vegetable fat blends and in some formulae partial replacement of fat with medium chain triglycerides (MCT) are used to enhance absorption. The latter should be regarded only as a source of energy as it neither contains, nor can it be metabolized to, essential fatty acid.

The feed osmolality should be as near that of human milk as possible (264 mmol/kg) in order to prevent osmolar diarrhoea, and optimalize absorption.

The exact nutritional needs of low birth weight infants vary with gestational age and birth weight as well as clinical condition. The optimal composition of preterm formulae feeds has not been established and new findings can be expected to lead to changes in recommendations continually. These formulae have a higher nutrient density to volume than modified milks. Some of the formulae (Table 1.6,**3**) currently available do not meet the recommendations already fairly well established, such as the protein considerations given above. Others are only intended for use in the short-term, for the very low birth weight infant.

FULL-TERM INFANTS WITH SPECIAL NEEDS

ADDITIONAL ENERGY

Failure to thrive, or respiratory and cardiac problems, in infants, may necessitate an increased energy intake. Additional feeds to increase intake should be advised in the first instance. In the breast-fed infant, additional suckling will stimulate milk production. The technique of feeding should be investigated to ensure proper suckling and latching on by the infant, so that the breast is properly emptied and the infant obtains the higher fat hind milk. In bottle-fed infants extra volume can be offered as an extra one or two feeds daily. Infants in hospital who will not willingly take extra volume or those requiring fluid restriction may benefit from high nutrient density feeds such as a suitable preterm type of formulae, e.g., Low Birth Weight SMA (J. Wyeth) (Table 1.6,**3**). Alternatively the simple addition of up to 3 g (1 level teaspoon) carbohydrate e.g., glucose polymer or sugar to each 100 ml of modified feed can supplement the energy intake provided the infant does not decrease his or her volume of feed to such an extent that protein and other nutrient intake becomes inadequate. The early introduction of weaning solids is appropriate in some infants, in order to increase total nutrient intake.

HABITUAL VOMITING AND HIATUS HERNIA

A thickened feed can be useful in reducing vomiting and the infant may benefit from being kept in a sitting position after feeds. Either 2 to 4 g starch (cornflour, arrowroot) or 0.5 to 1 g of a hemicellulose Nestargel (Nestlé) or Carobel (Cow & Gate) is cooked in each 100 ml water into which the milk powder is then incorporated. A regimen for the breast-fed infant is given on the Nestargel instruction sheet. These hemicellulose products give thickening without adding energy to the feed but may increase stool bulk. The carob seed from which they are made is thought to have a medicinal effect in reducing vomiting. Instant Carobel is now available as a pre-cooked thickener.

Bengers (Fisons Pharmaceuticals) is a mixture of amylase and trypsin enzymes in a wheat base with sodium bircarbonate. It is used to partially predigest the feed and increases the energy intake. It is inappropriate for the young infant in whom extra sodium and/or gluten are unsuitable. Usually 4% (weight to volume) Bengers is needed to thicken the feed, though up to 7 or 8% may be appropriate to increase the energy intake even further. The special instructions for preparation must be followed exactly to ensure maximum digestion and then to cook the starch.

Gaviscon (Reckitt & Coleman Pharmaceutical Division) is a gel of alginic acid, magnesium tricilicate, aluminium hydroxide and sodium bicarbonate in colloidal silica, and mannitol. It is used to control vomiting, does not require cooking but even the infant formula contains relatively large quantities of sodium (4 mmol per sachet) making it unsuitable for young infants or if sodium is contraindicated.

CONSTIPATION

Many mothers misinterpret straining at defaecation as constipation. Breast-fed infants may pass a stool every 10 days or 10 stools per day both of which are within the physiologically normal range. Constipation is rarely seen in the breast-fed infant. In the bottle-fed infant stools are usually passed at least on alternate days. Extra fluid, water or diluted fruit juice particularly natural or fresh orange juice is usually all that is needed to treat constipation in infants. Alternatively a spoonful of sugar (preferably brown) added to boiled water, fruit juice or one feed is a useful temporary means of correcting constipation. Once the infant is taking solids, fruit purées and cereals, and from 6 to 8 months of age wholegrain cereals such as Weetabix, should be encouraged.

GASTROENTERITIS

Breast-fed infants rarely get gastroenteritis. Oral rehydration fluids Dextrolyte (Cow & Gate), Dioralyte (Armour), Rehydrat (Searle) should be given but breast-feeding can continue. Bottle-fed infants should be given oral rehydration fluids for 24 hours then regraded quickly back onto appropriate feeds (Booth *et al.* 1984; Francis in press).

Table 1.9 Composition of DHSS Children's Vitamin A, D, C, Drops (Welfare Food Supplies).

5 drops contain		
	Vitamin A	200 μg
	Vitamin C	20 mg
	Vitamin D	7 μg (280 iu)

REDUCED FAT FEED

Infants are dependent on an adequate fat intake to provide their energy needs and human milk provides approximately 50% energy from fat. Normal infants have no need for a reduced fat feed and no commercial modified infant formulae are available in the UK because the fat of human milk and modern modified formulae containing a mixture of vegetable and animal fat are better absorbed than those with butterfat. The infant requiring a therapeutic reduced fat feed can often tolerate human milk, e.g., the infant with cystic fibrosis can be breast-fed although small quantities of pancreatin may be needed. Some 'follow-on' milks, e.g., Progress, contain only 2 g fat per 100 ml and can be introduced from the age of 6 months provided an adequate range and intake of weaning solids are taken by the infant.

VITAMIN SUPPLEMENTS FOR INFANTS AND CHILDREN

Exposure to sunlight on the skin produces vitamin D and is the major contribution to requirement. The Children's Vitamin A, D, C, Drops (Welfare Food Supplies) (5 drops per day) are recommended for all infants from about 1 month to 2 years and preferably 5 years of age unless the child is known to be getting an adequate alternative source of vitamins (DHSS 1983, revised). Table 1.9 gives details of their composition. The quantity of vitamins A and D in the standard dose of the Children's Vitamin A, D, C, Drops in addition to that contained in modified milks is still within safe limits for the majority of normal infants. Care should be taken that only one vitamin D supplement is given at any one time and the dose is measured carefully. Numerous commercial vitamin preparations are available.

WEANING: INTRODUCTION OF SOLIDS

Infants need a mixed diet when breast-feeding or when modified milk no longer provides adequate nutrition and development of feeding behaviour has progressed from sucking to biting and chewing. Solids should be given by spoon and not added to bottles. Solids should normally be commenced somewhere between 3 and 6 months of age (DHSS 1983, revised). Initially one item at a time is introduced. As solids are increased, feed volume should be reduced, and extra fluid offered as water, or diluted natural fruit juice. Demand feeds and solids according to appetite, allow the infant to dictate an appropriate intake for normal growth preventing in the majority both failure to thrive on the one hand, and obesity on the other. Energy to volume density is important (see p.12).

Initially a small quantity of fruit purées or a rice-based cereal mixed with part of the feed is commonly the first solid offered, e.g., Robinson's Baby Rice, Farex Weaning Food, Milupa Rice Cereal. New foods are introduced one at a time at 3- to 4-day intervals before a second then third feed. Salt should **not** be added or used in savoury foods given to young infants. Home prepared purées are suitable and considerably cheaper than commercial weaning foods, which have purely a convenience factor. Milk, egg, nuts, and pip fruits should be discouraged at least till 6 months of age in infants at risk of allergy (DHSS 1983, revised), and wheat is discouraged initially.

Iron-containing foods such as puréed liver or meat, green vegetables and iron-fortified cereals should be included. Egg yolk or scrambled egg is introduced at about 6 months of age in normal infants. Hard-boiled egg yolk is less sensitizing than soft-cooked egg, and the yolk is preferable to the white. Gradually additional tastes are added to each meal to expand variety.

A change to minced and mashed foods or junior foods between 6 and 9 months is important to get the infant used to new consistencies. A crust of bread and other finger foods should be offered (under supervision to avoid choking) to encourage chewing, which is also important for speech development. Breast-feeding can continue for as long as mother and infant want and there may be advantages in prolonged breast-feeding in those at risk of allergy (Saarinen *et al.* 1979). Breast-feeding or modified baby milks in decreasing quantity are ideally continued until 8 to 10 months when the infant is able to drink from a cup. In hospitals it is preferable to continue 'ready-to-feed' formulae for all bottle-fed infants, even into the second year as these are bacteriologically safer and the majority of sick children have an increased need for low solute modified milk.

Cow's milk, goat's milk and 'follow-on' milks should not be given before 6 months of age and are not recommended as bottle feeds. By about 10 to 12 months, bottles should be omitted and a change made to whole full fat cow's milk or 'follow-on' milk given from a cup or 'teacher beaker'. Approximately 500 ml milk and not more than 1000 ml per day is recommended. Reduced fat milks, skimmed milk and 'filled' milks should not be used for infants and young children. 'Follow-on' milks are higher in protein than modified milks and are fortified with iron and vitamins.

Natural wholegrain cereals and bread should be encouraged from 8 or 9 months but bran and fibre fortified foods are unnecessary and are not appropriate in the young child as the phytate content of cereal foods can inhibit trace mineral absorption. Due to the risk of inhalation whole nuts and hard sweets should not be given to young children.

A wide variety of high nutrient density foods in the diet selected

Table 1.10   Example menu for a young child or toddler.

On waking	Optional fruit juice (unsweetened)
Breakfast	Wholegrain cereal, Weetabix, porridge Whole full fat milk Wholemeal bread or toast, butter or margarine (PUFA)[a] Peanut butter, yeast extract, honey or marmalade Milk to drink Children's Vitamin A, D, C, Drops (Welfare Food Supplies) (plus Fluoride tablet/drops)
Mid-morning	Milk or fresh/natural fruit juice and/or piece of fruit
Lunch	Egg, cheese, baked beans, liver sausage, sardines, peanut butter Wholemeal bread and butter or margarine (PUFA)[a] Custard or yoghurt and/or fruit Water to drink
Tea	Minced or chopped meat dish, crisp grilled bacon, flaked fish or vegetarian dish including pulses Chopped or mashed potato and vegetables or skinned tomato Fruit, ice cream, custard, yoghurt or milk pudding **or** the family meal of suitable consistency **or** junior or toddler ready prepared baby food Milk to drink and/or small piece of cheese to finish the meal
Bedtime	Milk to drink

Lunch and tea are interchangeable

[a] **High in Poly Unsaturated Fatty Acids.**

from the food groups (Table 1.11) helps to ensure nutritional adequacy though no one food is essential. Table 1.10 provides a suggested toddler diet menu. Self-feeding usually by one year old and happy relaxed meal times without force-feeding or parental anxiety reduce the risk of food refusal which is particularly common during intercurrent infections when fluids can temporarily replace meals, and due to toddler independence when they are best ignored.

PREVENTION OF DENTAL CARIES

Continual snacking spoils the appetite for meals, contributes to constipation, and increases the risk of dental caries. However, young children often benefit from 3 small meals plus 2 to 3 snacks per day. Milk or cheese at the end of meals rather than sweets or biscuits reduces the risk of dental caries, and sugar should be used sparingly. Fluoridation of the water supply and the use of fluoride toothpaste has helped decrease the incidence of dental caries (Infirri 1984). In areas where this is not available supplements can be given. However, new reduced recommended levels have been suggested (*Lancet* Editorial, 1981).

0.25 mg fluoride from 2 weeks to 2 years old ⎫ where the fluoride
0.5 mg fluoride from 2 to 4 years old ⎬ level of water is
1 mg fluoride from 4 to 16 years old ⎭ 0.3 ppm

Where the fluoride level of water falls between 0.3 and 0.7 ppm, no supplement should be given until 2 years of age after which the recommended dose is halved.

THE DIETS OF CHILDREN

The nutritional state of an individual is dependent on the total food intake. Healthy children may include any available food in the diet as long as the total diet is satisfactory to promote growth, health and well-being and not excessive in those nutrients known to be toxic or to be deleterious to health. An infinite variety of food combinations can provide an adequate diet.

The nutrient density of the diet, that is the balance between energy and essential protective nutrients such as protein, vitamins,

Table 1.11 Food groups. (From Francis 1985.)

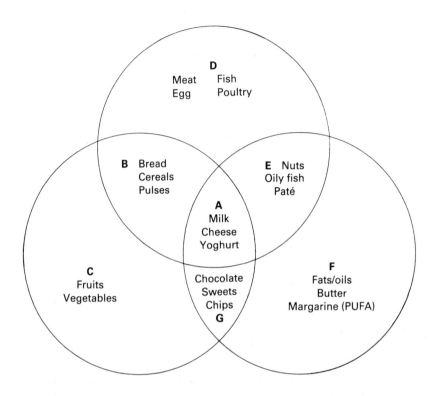

A Protein, calcium + vitamin B_2.

B Proteins, fibre and carbohydrates + B_1. (*Encourage to provide bulk of dietary intake*).

C Unrefined carbohydrates and fibre + vitamins A and C.

D Protein (low fat) with vitamin B, iron and zinc. (*1–2 serves daily.*)

E Proteins plus fats, alternatives to other protein foods. (*Use sparingly to reduce fat intake.*)

F Fats and oils. (*Use sparingly.*)

G Refined carbohydrates and fats. (*Avoid or limit.*)

minerals and fibre, is important to ensure the nutritional adequacy of the diet as a whole. Energy density to volume of food is also important (see p.12). Selection of foods from each food group daily (Table 1.11) together with the inclusion of as much variety of the different foods as possible helps to ensure the provision of a nutritionally adequate diet which meets the recommended nutrient intakes (Table 1.2).

No one food is indispensible so long as other foods from the same food group are included. However, milk is an important source of calcium, riboflavin and protein and therefore children under 5 years should normally be provided with 500 ml whole full fat milk or its equivalent per day, and those children who do not have milk, especially those under 2 years of age, should be supplied with a nutritionally adequate replacement in the form of a milk substitute, e.g., Wysoy (Table 1.6,**5**). Normally not more than 1000 ml milk per day is recommended. Older children for whom milk plays a diminishing nutritional role should be provided with at least 250 ml milk per day is recommended. Older children for whom milk plays a diminishing nutritional role should be provided with at least 250 ml milk per day, but it is optional as to whether it is skimmed, semi-skimmed or whole milk. Meat is an excellent source of vitamin B_{12}, absorbable iron and zinc and therefore makes a valuable contribution to the diet.

Many children under 5 years old have small appetites and they require an energy intake of less than 6700 kJ (1600 kcal) per day. They should be encouraged to have a diet with a high macro and micro nutrient density including energy. A wide range of basic foods including milk, cheese, wholemeal bread, lean meat, egg and fish, fruit and vegetables should be encouraged to provide the major dietary intake. Fats mostly as butter and/or fats high in polyunsaturated fatty acids should be included in moderation. The needs of the individual and the psychological-social aspects of eating must be kept in mind.

Similar principles apply to the older child as for the under 5-year-old. However, those families who elect to reduce dietary fat intake (unless the individual is overweight) must supply with physiological and acceptable sources of energy to replace the energy deficit normally supplied from fat. Table 1.12 gives one example of a menu for normal nutrition for school children. Table 1.13 gives a calculated example of a diet for a 5- to 7-year-old.

Table 1.12 Example menu for normal nutrition for school children.

Breakfast	Natural unsweetened fruit juice
	Wholegrain cereal, wheatflakes, cornflakes, porridge or muesli
	Milk or yoghurt
	Wholemeal bread or toast
	Butter or margarine (PUFA)[a]
	Optionals—egg, bacon (grilled), baked beans
	Marmite, Bovril, marmalade
	Tea, coffee, cocoa made with milk
Lunch/Dinner	School dinner **or**
	Wholemeal bread or rolls
	Margarine (PUFA)[a] or butter
	Various fillings, cheese, ham, egg, meat, fish or pâté, meat, pasta, peanut butter
	Salad or raw carrot, celery, tomato
	Fresh fruit, dried fruit, nuts, cheese
Snack after school	Fruit or sandwich, and glass of milk
Tea/Supper	Meat, fish, beans, lentils
	Potato, macaroni, rice and/or wholemeal bread
	or made up dish, e.g. pizza, risotto, fish pie, cottage pie, macaroni cheese
	Butter or margarine (PUFA)[a]
	Vegetables or salad
	Yoghurt, fruit, icecream or pudding
	Milk or cheese to finish the meal
Bedtime	Glass of milk (unsweetened) or tea, coffee, cocoa
	Older children may enjoy a bowl of cereal or a sandwich

[a] Poly Unsaturated Fatty Acids

Teenagers who require a high energy diet, especially if in excess of 14 000 kJ (3300 kcal) per day normally obtain adequate nutrients even if their density falls below average. However, very high energy intakes require a high energy density to volume, and the fat, sugar and fibre intakes may need to be in excess of the recommendations given by NACNE (James 1983) and the *Diet and Cardiovascular Disease* (DHSS 1984) reports. The so-called 'empty calorie' foods are more acceptable and help keep the cost of the diet within practical limits (Passmore *et al.* 1979).

Diets in Ethnic Groups

A number of racial groups have dietary restrictions for cultural or religious reasons (DHSS 1981b). The adequacy of these diets requires scrutiny to ensure they are appropriate for optimal growth in children. The diets which inhibit the use of only a few foods or food combinations can provide adequate nutrition which compares favourably with Western traditional diets. However, severely limited diets such as macrobiotic and fruitarian diets are unsuitable as they do not provide adequate nutrients for growth (Roberts et al. 1979).

Changes in traditional eating patterns occur in immigrants due to the lack of availability of certain foods, their cost and the lack of knowledge about suitable alternatives and their preparation. The resultant diet may be nutritionally inadequate.

Sunlight exposure on skin can provide adequate vitamin D. This may be inadequate in northern cities and cold climates which interfere with irradiation, or where infants are swaddled or kept indoors with mothers confined by the purdah system. Rickets can result. Asians in Britain have a higher incidence of rickets and osteomalacia (DHSS 1980b). The reason for this has received considerable attention, particularly as dietary vitamin D intake does not appear to differ from non-immigrant groups, sunlight exposure has not been found to be less, and skin pigmentation does not appear to be related. However, the intake of high extraction cereal diets as used in chappatis and unleavened bread in which calcium binding occurs is related to the low vitamin D status. The exact cause of the calcium binding is not clear (Burman & McLaren 1982), but may be related to the phytate content of the diet. Vitamin D supplements can prevent these diseases and are now recommended to be taken by Asians living in Britain throughout childhood, adolescence, in pregnancy, and lactation, and for all children until at least 2 years old.

The commonest cultural and religious diets are:

1. **Kosher.** Jews exclude pork, rabbit, shellfish, eels etc. Meat must be ritually slaughtered (Kosher). Milk and its products and meat must not be taken in the same meal. During Passover no leavened bread is permitted.

2. **Halal.** Moslems exclude pork and all forms of carnivorous animals. Alcohol is forbidden. Meat is ritually slaughtered (Halal).

3. **Hindus** and **sikhs** usually exclude beef and pork, and are frequently ova vegetarians who will take milk. Strict dietary laws

Table 1.13 Calculated example of a diet for a school child of 5 to 7 years old.

	Edible weight food g	Energy kcal	Energy kJ	Protein g	Fat g	Carbohydrate g
Breakfast						
Cereal, e.g. Weetabix	30	102	433	3.4	0.6	15
Sugar	5	20	84	—	—	5
Wholemeal bread	50	108	459	4.4	0.5	25
Butter or margarine (PUFA)[a]	10	74	304	Trace	8.0	—
Peanut butter	10	62	258	2.3	3.0	5
Marmite, Bovril, Yeastil, honey or marmalade	—	≈30	≈120	Trace	—	5
Milk (± tea/coffee)	200 ml	130	544	6.6	7.2	10
Mid-morning snack						
Fruit, e.g. orange	120	42	180	1.0	—	10
Lunch/Dinner						
Meat—beef stew	50	60	249	5.4	6.0	—
Potato—mashed or jacket	100	119	499	1.5	—	20
Vegetables—carrots and/or sprouts	50	10[b]	39[b]	1.0[a]	—	3[b]
Fruit crumble	50	104	439	0.9	1.1	20
Custard (with powder)	30	35	149	1.1	1.1	5

Tea/Snack						
Crisps	20	107	445	1.3	6.7	10
Supper/Packed lunch						
Baked beans (canned)	100					
or						
Egg, boiled	50	86[b]	355[b]	6.0[b]	4.0[b]	10[b]
or						
Fish fingers, fried	50					
Wholemeal bread	100	216	918	8.8	1.0	50
Butter or margarine (PUFA)[a]	20	148	608	Trace	8.0	—
Fruit, e.g. apple	150	69	294	0.5	—	10
Milk (± tea/coffee)	200 ml	130	544	6.6	7.2	10
Total		1652	6921	50.8 12% energy	70.4 38% energy	213 52% energy

[a] Poly Unsaturated Fatty Acids
[b] Average

apply during special religious festivals and fasting is often a feature.

4.   **Vegetarianism** occurs in people of every country and creed. Meat is excluded as no flesh, fish or fowl is eaten. Lacto ova vegetarians also exclude milk and egg. Lacto vegetarians also exclude milk but permit egg. Ova vegetarians also exclude egg but permit milk.

5.   **Vegans** exclude all animal products, i.e., meat, egg, honey. Pulse and cereal combinations are necessary in order to provide adequate protein of high biological value. The cooking of cereals and soaking and cooking of pulses makes them more digestible. A nutritionally adequate diet can be devised using the Vegan Society dietary principles. Energy density of such diets is however frequently low and can result in failure to thrive as young children cannot always consume an adequate volume of food for their energy needs. Vegan children tend to be smaller than their peers. Infants should be breast-fed, then weaned onto a nutritionally adequate soya modified milk such as Cow & Gate S Formula. A supplement of 1 to 2 mg vitamin B_{12} must be given as it is not obtainable from plant sources. Folic acid is largely destroyed by the long slow cooking process used for cereals and pulses and therefore fresh vegetables should be included. Iron and calcium must be provided by inclusion of unrefined cereals and pulses, seeds and dark green leaf vegetables rich in these minerals; calcium-rich foods include ragi (finger millet) and sesame seeds; iron-rich foods include teff and mung beans and some seaweeds; the latter also provide iodine.

Meat has zinc and iron of high bioavailability whereas a vegan diet is high in phytate which inhibits the availability of zinc, calcium and iron, therefore, the exclusion of meat necessitates a generous intake of foods high in these minerals.

Vitamin A is provided as provitamin carotene from plant foods especially those of the dark green and yellow type; carrots, apricots and red palm oil are excellent sources.

Vitamin D acquired from exposure to sunlight in this country is frequently inadequate and should be provided from supplements or dietary sources such as a suitable fortified margarine, e.g. Tomor (Van den Bergh) or Tela (Israeli Foods) Kosher margarines which are also milk-free and solely of vegetable sources. They can also be used or combined in equal proportions with butter for ghee to provide a more adequate vitamin D intake in Asian diets.

Table 1.14 Examples of a vegan diet for children of different ages.

A suitable nutritionally adequate soya milk substitute should be encouraged, e.g. Cow & Gate S Formula.

1 Weaning/toddler diet

Breakfast	Cereal and soya milk substitute Wholemeal bread or toast and kosher margarine Yeast extract Natural fruit juice
Lunch	Purée or mashed pulses (soaked, cooked and skins removed) **or** 1–2 teaspoons peanut butter Cooked cereal, e.g. wholegrain rice or pasta Dark green and other vegetables Fruit and/or soya custard
Snacks	Soya milk substitute Fruit
Tea	Lentil and barley soup Wholemeal bread and kosher margarine Peanut butter or yeast extract Fruit
Supper	Soya milk substitute

2 Older child

Breakfast	Cereal and soya milk substitute Wholemeal bread or toast or kosher margarine Peanut butter, yeast extract Natural fruit juice
Lunch	Nutmeat or vegetarian dish containing pulses Vegetables or salad Wholegrain pasta or rice or wholemeal bread and kosher margarine Fruit
Supper	Vegetarian dish containing cereal and pulses or nutmeat Dark green vegetables Rice, pasta or wholemeal bread and kosher margarine Soya milk substitute Fruit
Snacks	Fruit and nuts and/or muesli or sesame seed bar Wholewheat crisps

6. **Zen macrobiotic diets** are based on unrefined cereals frequently excluding or limiting vegetables and fruits and limiting fluid intake. Although no food is actually forbidden food combinations are very important. Fruitarian diets are based on

fruit and fermented, but uncooked, cereals and seeds. These diets are nutritionally inadequate to support normal growth in young children; protein energy malnutrition, anaemia and vitamin deficiency have been reported (Roberts et al. 1979). Such diets should be discouraged in children.

Infants are frequently breast-fed by these cultural groups. Weaning solids should be introduced at the normal age and not later than 8 months in order to prevent growth failure and anaemia occurring. Non-breast-fed infants and pre-school age children from those groups who exclude cow's milk from the diet should be encouraged to use a nutritionally adequate non-animal product such as soya milk, S Formula or Granolac Infant (Granose). Vegans, vegetarians, Moslems and Jews will not accept products such as SMA, Progress or Wysoy which contain oleo oil from beef fat, and Prosobee which contains traces of gelatine used to suspend some of the vitamins. Premium (Cow & Gate) and Osterfeed (Farley) which do not contain animal products except milk, are accepted by vegetarian, Moslem and Jewish families.

An example of a weaning and older child's vegan diet menu is given in Table 1.14. An excess intake of fruit juices, wholegrain foods and pulses can lead to diarrhoea and should be avoided particularly if it results in growth failure.

Useful sources of dietary information in devising diets for various cultural groups are given at the end of this chapter, as are the addresses of the various societies who will provide advice about their racial or cultural diets.

Protein Energy Malnutrition and Failure to Thrive

Protein energy malnutrition is a common problem of nutrition particularly affecting young children in the third world. It is inter-related with gastroenteritis and other infections to which the malnourished child is prone and they in their turn lead to malnutrition. McLaren (1982b), Hansen et al. (1982), and Cameron & Hofvander (1983) give details of the condition, prevention and treatment, and the latter gives detailed recipes and feeds using locally available foods. Specific deficiencies, e.g., dehydration, vitamin A deficiency and anaemia should be corrected as a matter of urgency. The dietary regimen devised for rehabilitation should be nutritionally adequate, and should be started as soon as possible. Initially a regimen based on whole milk fortified with the addition of 5% carbohydrate and 2% fat is fed at 150 ml/kg per day.

Vitamin and mineral supplements including multivitamins, folic acid, vitamin A, iron and potassium should be given. Hypothermia and hypoglycaemia are common. Feeds should be given during the day and night and the child kept warm, especially initially. To allow for catch-up growth, 2 to 3 g protein and possibly 4 g protein with 630 to 840 kJ (150 to 200 kcal)/kg per day should be provided after the first few days and gradually locally available foods should replace the milk feeds.

Mild protein energy malnutrition occurs more widely, also happening in the Western world, especially in economically deprived social groups, toddlers and children weaned onto inappropriate diets, and chronically ill children of all ages, e.g., those with cardiac disease. Inadequate energy intake for whatever cause, results in poor growth and the use of protein for energy needs. Other nutritional deficiencies occur simultaneously ·and may of themselves lead to failure to thrive, e.g., zinc deficiency or indirectly anaemia leading to poor appetite. Prevention through education programmes and an adequate food supply is of paramount importance.

ANOREXIA AND FOOD REFUSAL

Energy density must be increased if the child is unable to manage the bulk of food needed for energy needs. Fat and sugars are useful sources of energy in the diet which can increase energy density. Additional opportunities to eat, e.g., 3 meals plus 2 to 3 snacks per day allows the child's intake to increase.

Force-feeding should be avoided though patience and encouragement may be necessary. Correction of underlying disease and deficiency often results in clinical improvement, an improved appetite, and resultant increased intake. A variety of foods can be used to tempt jaded appetites such as ice-cream, milk shakes, etc.

Toddler food refusal is so common it can be thought of as part of normal development and the need to be independent (see Introduction, p.1). Most of these children are of normal weight despite the bizarre or inadequate diet described by parents who can become intensely anxious. The parents should be reassured and the food strikes ignored as they are short-lived if not permitted to become a battleground and an attention-seeking device. A detailed dietary history, including information about the atmosphere surrounding meals, usually reveals the problem. The child should be offered food and allowed to eat to appetite without forcing or comment. Snack foods are usually more acceptable than traditional meals. Parents and professionals with idealistic ideas of nutrition need to accept that a child can live temporarily on a diet of crisps, chocolate, milk and fruit juice. Whole milk should be offered, though excess quantity (more than 1000 ml (35 oz) per day) should be discouraged and energy supplements such as glucose polymers are inapproriate as they only satisfy the appetite without encouraging the child to take a proper diet. Bentovim (1970) found that as many as 30% of 4-year-olds, when the peak incidence is reached, are finicky eaters existing on bizarre diets. If parental anxiety continues the eating pattern can become an attention-seeking device.

ANOREXIA NERVOSA

Anorexia nervosa (see also Introduction, p.4) is a psychiatric syndrome consisting of a severe state of malnutrition by self-imposed starvation in association with a changed perception of the body image and fear of normal weight. It has similarities to the 'hunger strikes' of infants and toddlers but commonly occurs in adolescent girls and young women. The incidence has increased in the last decade, and it tends to occur in those from middle class families where food is plentiful, and where sometimes obesity is present in other family members or in the patient at an earlier age. The diagnosis and clinical features have been well described by Crisp (1977) and Norton (1983). Many different treatment programmes exist usually including refeeding and psychotherapy simultaneously. The aim of dietetic treatment is to get the patient to eat and to gain weight. A normal diet for age is appropriate but needs modification for the patient's preferences but it is unrealistic to expect a patient to eat a full diet at once. Some patients may require enteral or parenteral nutrition in the first instance. One therapist, usually the psychiatrist, must be in charge of the patient and should be prepared to follow up the patient over a long period of time. The dietitian's role is to provide nutritional information and an appropriate diet but she or he should not get involved in the food manipulations and bargaining about food which the patient inevitably tries to precipitate. These patients are intelligent and usually have an excellent knowledge of nutrition.

Outcome for the individual is dependent upon personal, environmental and treatment factors all of which interact. The disease can be a mild transitory state which may remit or a chronic severe illness. Maintenance of a 'normal' body weight alone does not signify a cure. One third of recognized sufferers may not benefit from treatment and of those who show improvement a proportion live what appears to be an unnecessarily restricted and empty life.

Vitamin and Mineral Deficiencies

Major deficiencies of vitamins and minerals are rare in normal children in this country (see Chapter 3). They can occur in specific susceptible groups such as toddlers from immigrant groups, patients in long-stay hospitals, those on various cult diets, in association with protein energy malnutrition, or children on inadequate therapeutic regimens.

Anaemia may occur particularly in toddlers who live on milk, in those in whom weaning is delayed or where there is difficulty in getting the child on to solids and some vegetarians. Other nutritional deficiencies may be present. Inadequate iron, folic acid and/or vitamin B_{12} are responsible. Liver, meat, dark green vegetables, unrefined and fortified cereals and egg yolk are all sources of iron and B vitamins. Vitamin C given at the same meal, e.g., as fruit juice enhances iron absorption.

Anaemia is relatively common in immigrant groups whose traditional diet makes no provision for weaning foods (Jivani 1978). Adequate practical advice regarding appropriate weaning foods which are acceptable to the cultural diet is essential. Foods rich in iron and calcium should be encouraged; for example, cereals such as ragi (finger millet) and sesame seeds are rich in calcium; bajra (spiked millet) is a good source of iron as are legumes, dark green leafy vegetables and mung beans. Vitamin B_{12} is not found in plant food so vegetarians should be given supplements. The modified soya formulae (Table 1.6,**5**), but not all soya milks, are fortified with calcium and vitamins including vitamin B_{12} (*Drugs and Therapeutics Bulletin*, Editorial, 1983). Folic acid and vitamins C and B_{12} are destroyed in the traditional long slow cooking employed in making curry and those following the principles of Zen macrobiotics. The latter frequently exclude fruit, so scurvy as well as anaemia can occur.

The excessive use of refined carbohydrate to replace traditional foods reduces the intake of zinc, calcium, iron and other trace minerals (Underwood 1977). Convenience foods and changing food habits are altering the intake of the leser known trace nutrients. A wide range of natural foods including fruit, vegetables, some red meat and a generous intake of wholegrain cereals to provide a nutrient dense diet is the best protection from dietary inadequacy.

Vitamin Toxicity

The increasing fashion for 'health foods' and supplements increases the risk of vitaminosis. Excessive, unphysiological quantities are often given. This is both wasteful and unnecessary provided the diet is adequate (see Chapter 3 for further details). An excess intake of carrots, green vegetables, apricots etc. can lead to caratenaemia with characteristic yellow pigmentation of the palms of the hands. This is easily diagnosed compared to vitamin A poisoning which has a whole range of symptoms and is only revealed by a dietary history including supplements. Caratenaemia is occasionally seen in young children and can be a feature of anorexia nervosa and those on fruitarian and vegetarian diets. Though harmless a reduction of the carotene containing fruit and vegetables (apricots and carrots) is advised.

Hypercalcaemia due to vitamin D overdose is now rare, except in those who appear to have a predisposition and acquire idiopathic hypercalcaemia even on normal intakes of vitamin D (DHSS 1980b). The latter is more fully dealt with by Francis (in press).

Water-soluble vitamins taken in excess of needs are excreted in the urine and toxicity is unlikely.

There is a current tendency to take huge doses of vitamin C (ascorbic acid) to prevent the common cold and reduce the risk of heart disease; only a small proportion is absorbed. This practice can result in vitamin C addiction, renal calculi and even renal tubular damage has occurred with doses of several gram per day taken over a long period. Urinary oxalate is increased with high doses of vitamin C in some subjects (Hughes *et al.* 1981). A generous intake from natural fruit and vegetable sources is recommended (e.g., 100 mg per day). Supplements of 250 mg ascorbic acid are harmless when given for several days at the first signs of an intercurrent infection and may enhance recovery. Doses of 1 gram or more per day, especially when taken long-term, should be discouraged.

ACUTE INFECTIONS AND CATABOLISM

Even minor intercurrent infections cause loss of appetite and in young children are often accompanied by diarrhoea and vomiting. It is important to prevent dehydration with adequate fluids or oral rehydration solutions (Booth *et al.* 1984). Temporary reduction in nutrient intake apart from fluid and electrolytes is insignificant in the majority of well-nourished children, but after the infection nutrient losses must be made up to allow for catch-up growth. Usually the child's appetite is the best guide provided he or she is given ample opportunity to eat.

The parents of chronically ill children need guidance about intake, replacements and a list of priorities regarding different foods to offer in order to prevent chronic growth failure. This is particularly important if the child is on a therapeutic diet in which nutrient intake is restricted.

Catabolic States and the Severely Ill Child

Children and particularly infants have far fewer body reserves of all nutrients including energy than have adults (Heird *et al.* 1972). As a result they can only withstand very short periods of starvation before death will occur (Table 1.15). During starvation initially glycogen stores are used, then fat and later protein to provide essential energy for basal metabolism. This energy is required by different organs of the body for the proportion needed by each varies with the weight of the patient. A 5 kg child for example requires approximately 65% of his or her basal metabolic energy for brain metabolism, 18% for liver, 8% for muscle and the remainder

Table 1.15 Energy reserves during starvation in different aged children compared to adults. (Adapted from Heird *et al.* 1972.)

	Energy reserve[a]		Estimated number of days for total depletion of energy reserves	
	kJ/kg	kcal/kg	Starvation	Partial starvation[b]
Small preterm infant	840	200	5	10
Large preterm infant	2500	600	12	32
Term infant	6700	1600	32	75
1-year-old child	9200	2200	42	110
Adult	7950	1900	90	400

[a] Non protein energy + ⅓ protein energy.

[b] Partial starvation as represented by 5% dextrose supplying fluid needs.

remainder for other organs; a 20 kg child needs about 42% of his or her basal metabolic energy for brain metabolism, 25% for liver, 13% for muscle and the remainder for other organs; but an adult in comparison needs about 25% for each organ (Heird *et al.* 1972). Starvation and clinical situations which use body reserves are therefore much more critical in children than in adults and in the infant compared to older children. The primary aim is to provide essential energy for basal metabolism, secondly to stop catabolism and correct nutritional deficiencies and then thirdly, to reverse catabolism to anabolism. In the anabolic phase, requirements may be much higher than normal.

Illness and tissue repair impose additional demands on nutritional supply and the activity of body defence mechanisms may also increase nutritional need. Metabolic changes occur with increased urinary nitrogen losses proportional to the severity of the illness (Cuthbertson 1980). A summary of the changes in adult resting metabolic rates is given in Figure 1.2 (Elwyn 1980).

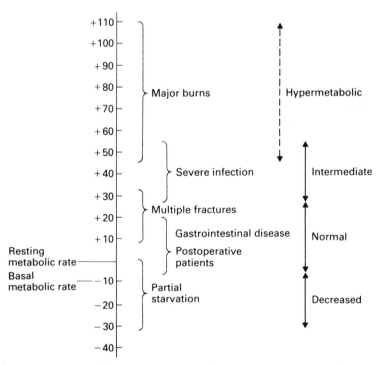

Fig. 1.2 Percentage change in resting metabolic rate in different clinical conditions in adults. (From Elwyn 1980.)

Severe injury causes negative nitrogen balance and weight loss which cannot be prevented at the time of stress (Richards 1977). In the hypercatabolic patient glycogen stores are depleted, fat breakdown occurs causing ketosis, and is not reversed by giving glucose. Glyconeogenesis and glucose oxidation also occur at increased rates due to catabolic hormonal changes associated with the 'stress' response (Grant & Todd 1982). New protein synthesis is depressed and the rate of protein breakdown is increased (James 1981). Protein depletion, sodium metabolic changes and potassium loss occur. Secondary nutritional deficiencies such as anaemia, vitamin deficiency and trace mineral depletion can subsequently result. Adequate fluid intake and energy for basal metabolic rate is of prime importance with maintenance of electrolyte homeostasis. Infections should be treated rigorously. Severe catabolism with large nutrient losses results in poor wound healing, lethargy, anorexia, and increased risk of infection. Adequate intake of energy minimizes nitrogen losses and action should be taken to replenish nutrient loss. Nitrogen balance in seriously ill hypermetabolic patients can be improved by administering glucose and exogenous insulin to maintain normoglycaemia (Woolfson *et al.* 1979).

Burman (1982) gives a guide to estimate the extent of protein catabolism:

g/24 hours urinary urea × 3.6 if blood urea is constant;
g/24 hours urinary urea × 3.6 plus rise in blood urea (g/litre) × 1.8
× kg body weight if the blood urea is rising.

Such losses should be replaced with approximately 840 kJ (200 kcal) together with each 1 g nitrogen, i.e., approximately 135 kJ (32 kcal) with each 1 g protein.

Other losses should be estimated and methods of assessment are described by Grant & Todd (1982).

The child's weight together with clinical assessment of the state of hydration will give an assessment of nutritional status and fluid needs. Plasma and urinary electrolytes should be measured daily and intake and output charts should be used to record fluid, protein (nitrogen), sodium and potassium, energy intake and the weight of the child.

NUTRIENT NEEDS IN THE SEVERELY ILL CHILD

Nutritional requirements in the anabolic phase of illness are elevated compared to normal. Adequate intake of all nutrients, including vitamins and trace minerals is essential (Bunker & Clayton 1983). However, estimates of intakes can only be approximate and therefore clinical and biochemical monitoring with adjustment of intake appropriately should be used to ensure that each patient's requirements are met. Both energy and protein adjustments may be needed to maintain a positive nitrogen balance. Generally basal requirements for protein and energy should be increased in accordance with estimated or actual increase in metabolic rate (see Figure 1.2) or severity of injury. For example, energy intake in severe infections is in the range of 30 to 50% higher than normal and 50% up to 100% above normal in severe burns. Protein intake is similarly increased, but if too much is given, the blood urea can rise. An intake of 4 g/kg per day or twice the normal protein requirement on a weight basis is adequate except in patients with major burns or conditions causing major protein losses such as protein-losing enteropathy, nephrotic syndrome or skin conditions, e.g., acrodematitis bulosa. In patients with burns the Sutherland (1976) formula can be used to calculate nutritional needs. The intake must be adjusted for age in children, with an average of:

$$\begin{array}{lll} 3\text{ g protein per kg} & 250\text{ kJ per kg} & \left(\begin{array}{l}60\text{ kcal per kg}\\ +35\text{ kcal per }\%\text{ burn}\end{array}\right)\\ +1\text{ g per }\%\text{ burn} & +145\text{ kJ per }\%\text{ burn} & \end{array}$$

Great care must be taken when monitoring the intake in infants who have a lower margin of tolerance both for excess as well as inadequate intake.

Adequate fluid and electrolytes are essential. Gastrointestinal losses due to gastroenteritis, short gut syndrome, an ileostomy or colostomy must be corrected. In burns and skin conditions fluid and electrolyte losses through the skin must also be replenished. Feeding actually increases water requirement because more urine is produced to excrete waste products and the total volume of feed is not the total fluid available, e.g., 100 ml milk = 87 ml free fluid.

Carbohydrate and fat can both be used to supply the energy needs. Fat alone is ineffective at inhibiting protein breakdown for gluconeogenesis, but with some glucose it appears as effective at maintaining a positive nitrogen balance as glucose alone. To prevent ketosis, it is recommended that carbohydrate intake should always exceed that of fat and roughly an equal quantity of energy from both is recommended (Elwyn 1980).

At least in infants and patients on enteral feeds, the osmolality of the feed should be as near that of blood (approximately 300 mmol/kg) as possible and should not exceed 500 mmol/kg. High concentrations of carbohydrate increase the osmolality of the feed to unacceptable levels and can precipitate diarrhoea. The quantity of nutrients in each 100 ml of feed is a guide to the amount tolerated and the final osmolality of the feed, though the latter also depends on the choice of ingredients. Glucose polymers are lower in osmolality than monosaccharides, as is whole protein lower than peptides and amino acids, and long chain dietary fats and oils lower than medium chain triglycerides (MCT) for the same percentage solution. The following is a guide to the concentrations tolerated in enteral feeds used as the sole source of nutrition for paediatric patients over 2 years old:

10 to 12 g carbohydrate in each 100 ml (% weight/volume) up to a maximum of 15%

4 to 5 g fat in each 100 ml (% weight/volume) up to a maximum of 7%

2 to 3.5 g protein in each 100 ml (% weight/volume) up to a maximum of 4%

2 to 3 mmol sodium in each 100 ml up to a maximum of 7.7 mmol in each 100 ml

Approximately 420 kJ (100 kcal) in each 100 ml up to a maximum of 630 kJ (150 kcal) in each 100 ml

Osmolality ideally 280 to 350 mmol/kg and a maximum 500 mmol/kg. Under 2-year-olds usually tolerate the lower concentrations, older children may tolerate the higher concentrations.

Vitamin and minerals including trace elements should be provided to meet the individual's requirements (Aggett & Davies 1983) which may be slightly above normal (see Chapter 3). Appropriate supplements should be prescribed, if the selected feed does not contain an adequate range or quantity in the volume ingested. Vitamin-Mineral Supplement Tablets (Cow & Gate) plus Ketovite liquid (Paines & Byrne) provide a comprehensive range of vitamins and trace minerals and the dose can be tailored to the individual's needs and the contribution from the selected feed or food sources.

CHOICE OF FEEDING THE SICK CHILD

A patient who will not spontaneously take adequate nutrition from traditional foods should be encouraged to have an increased intake by offering extra snacks and drinks. Many children will willingly eat crisps, sandwiches, cereals, biscuits, cakes, chocolate and drinks including milk shakes, fortified fruit juices and carbonated beverages. Soup and savoury snacks may be preferred to sweet food, e.g., egg on toast, baked beans and meat burgers or fish fingers, and of course, chips are always popular. Savoury Complan (Farley) is now available. Small frequent snacks of these foods may suffice in providing an adequate intake. The dietitian should assess the intake and encourage the provision of a selection of appropriate items. Reassurance to parents and medical colleagues is often necessary as these foods are considered junk food and their value, particularly in short-term situations, is often underestimated. The child should be encouraged to eat to appetite; praise and reward should be used and reprimands are not appropriate. Supplements can be prescribed to make up deficit energy, protein, vitamins and minerals. Drinks are a particularly useful way of increasing intake and can be fortified with glucose polymers, skimmed milk powder, ice-cream or made up from commercially available products. Grant & Todd (1982) give some useful fortified drink recipes, and some examples suitable for children over 2 years are given in Table 1.16. The younger children could be given half quantities. These recipes are intended to be used in conjunction with other food and fluids, and should not be used as the sole source of nutrition. A high protein intake without adequate total energy will result in the protein being used as an expensive source of energy, and the blood urea will rise. Energy intake without adequate protein will not totally prevent nitrogen losses; protein depletion and nutritional inadequacy of other nutrients is common.

FLUID DIETS, ENTERAL FEEDS AND SUPPLEMENTS

Infants and young children require individual assessment of their nutritional needs. Extra volume of an appropriate modified formula (Table 1.6) is frequently all that is necessary. However:

1.   The higher protein modified milks may be preferable in some situations, e.g., Milumil (Milupa), Baby Milk Plus (Cow & Gate).

2.   Some of the 'preterm' formulae, e.g., Low Birth Weight SMA (Table 1.6,3) are a useful alternative to modified formulae as they have a higher density of protein, energy and other nutrients compared to volume. Osterprem is inappropriate in these circumstances due to its very high vitamin D content.

3.　A carefully calculated increase in concentration of feed can also be used, e.g., 15% dilution Gold Cap SMA (J. Wyeth) (4 scoops per 100 ml), compared to the normal 13% reconstitution, contains 1.8 g protein 320 kJ (77 kcal) in each 100 ml and is tolerated by many infants.

4.　Alternatively 3 g carbohydrate can be added to each 100 ml of most modified formulae, particularly if a glucose polymer (or sugar) is used to increase the carbohydrate content to approximately 10 g and the energy content to 323 kJ (77 kcal) in each 100 ml. It is essential to ensure adequate volume of feed is taken to meet the protein requirement.

5.　A follow-on milk, e.g., Progress (Table 1.6,**4**) may be appropriate as it has a higher protein content than modified milks, and is fortified with iron and vitamins.

For the child who cannot eat and for whom semi-solids and supplements alone still do not provide adequate intake due to illness, facial injury or unconsciousness, a fluid diet (Table 1.17) is required; either fed orally or as an enteral tube feed. The psychological effect of a fluid diet in a child who is conscious is important. Normal food, e.g., ice-cream which can easily be incorporated into a feed can boost the morale and can be important to the child who is unable to eat or has only 'sham' feeds. The child who enjoys seeing, and smelling, food can have his or her meal served out like others in the family even if it then has to be liquidized to be fed as a fluid, by gastrostomy or nasogastric or nasojejunal tube. Care over palatability, variety, colour and odour is needed for fluid diets, especially if taken by mouth. Strained baby foods can be useful additives, but need to be balanced by fortified drinks and supplements (Tables 1.16 & 1.17) to ensure the total intake is nutritionally adequate. Variety also helps overcome the risk of trace nutrient deficiency. However, vitamin and trace nutrient supplements should be prescribed if there is doubt regarding the nutritional adequacy of the intake.

Enteral feeds should preferably be given as small frequent (2-hourly) cyclical feeds which more closely mimic normal feeding patterns than continuous feeds and they are better absorbed than large bolus feeds. They also allow the child more freedom for play and social activities. They are also safer in that fluid overload is less likely to occur provided the bolus feed is measured and calculated appropriately for the child's age and weight and there is less fear of the tube becoming displaced with subsequent feed inhalation. However, continuous feeds can be useful in patients requiring large

Table 1.16 Fortified drinks and supplements for children over 2 years of age.

	Energy		Carbohydrate	Protein	Fat
	kJ	kcal	g	g	g
1 200 ml milk[d]	544	130	9.4	6.6	7.6
20 g skimmed milk powder	300	72	10.6	7.2	0.2
Total =	844	202	20.0	13.8	7.8
2 200 ml milk[d]	544	130	9.4	6.6	7.6
40 g ice-cream (dairy)	280	66	10.0	1.4	2.6
Total =	824	196	19.4	8.0	10.2
3 200 ml milk[d]	544	130	9.4	6.6	7.6
20 g Complan (Farley)	374	88	11.0	4.0	3.2
Total =	918	218	20.4	10.6	10.8
4 200 ml milk[d]	544	130	9.4	6.6	7.6
7 g Casilan (Farley) / **or** 7 g Maxipro (SHS) }[e]	105	25	Trace	6.3	0.2
10 g Nesquick or equivalent flavouring	160	40	10.0	Trace	Trace
Total =	809	195	19.4	13.9	7.8
5 200 ml milk[d]	544	130	9.4	6.6	7.6
25 g Build-Up (Carnation)	363	87	17.0	5.6	0.3
Total =	907	217	26.4	12.2	7.9
6 150 ml (approx) tomato soup (ready-to-serve) }[ce]	345	83	8.9	1.2	5.0
30 g skimmed milk powder }	450	108	15.9	10.8	0.3
Water to 200 ml	—	—	—	—	—
Total =	795	191	24.8	12.0	5.3
7 1 egg[a]	306	73	Trace	6.1	5.5
150 ml fresh or natural orange juice[b]	242	57	14.1	0.9	Trace
5 g glucose polymer	80	20	5.0	—	—
Total =	628	150	19.1	7.0	5.5

8	100 g fruit yoghurt[d]	405	95	17.9	4.8	1.0
	100 ml milk[d]	272	65	4.7	3.3	3.8
		Total = 677	160	22.6	8.1	4.8
9	1 banana (100 g)[b]	337	79	19.2	1.1	0.3
	150 ml milk[d]	408	98	7.1	5.0	5.7
	10 g double cream	184	45	0.2	0.2	4.8
		Total = 929	222	26.5	6.3	10.8
10	40 g ice-cream (dairy)	280	66	10.0	1.4	2.6
	Add just before drinking: 25 ml undiluted Ribena and water to 150 ml or 150 ml CocaCola } or 150 ml lemonade } + 7 g glucose polymer[e]	250	58	15.4	Trace	—
		Total = 530	124	25.4	1.4	2.6
11	100 g fruit yoghurt	405	95	17.9	4.8	1.0
	20 g double cream	368	90	0.4	0.4	9.6
	10 g glucose polymer	160	40	10.0	Trace	—
	Water may be added to 200 ml					
		Total = 993	225	28.3	5.2	10.6
12	100 ml tomato soup } (ready-to-serve, canned)[c,e]	230	55	5.9	0.8	3.3
	100 g baked beans }	270	64	10.3	5.1	0.5
	(puréed)	Total = 500	119	16.2	5.9	3.8

[a] Raw egg white contains avidin which binds biotin from the yolk, making it unavailable. More than one raw egg should not be given in any one day. [b] High in potassium. [c] High in sodium.
[d] Normally whole fat milk is recommended but Channel Island (gold top) milk can be used and is higher in energy and fat content. [e] Average.

The ingredients should normally be homogenized and served chilled. Savoury recipes can be heated. Many children can be encouraged to take these recipes if given them with a drinking straw or if they are served in cartoons similar to those used by commercial cafeterias.

These recipes are intended to be used in conjunction with other foods and drinks and not as the sole source of nutrition.

Table 1.17 Fluid diet examples for children of different ages.

	Energy		Carbohydrate	Protein	Fat
	kJ	kcal	g	g	g
1 2- to 4-year old					
500 ml milk (whole full fat)	1360	325	23.5	16.5	19.0
50 g glucose polymer and/or flavouring	800	200	50.0	Trace	—
10 ml Prosparol/Calogen/double cream	184	45	0.2	0.2	4.8
200 ml fruit juice – natural orange juice	323	76	19.0	1.2	—
20 g glucose polymer	335	80	20.0	—	—
150 ml tomato soup (ready-to-serve)	345	83	9.0	1.2	5.0
Banana Milk Shake (Table 1.16, 9)	929	222	26.5	6.3	10.8
Yoghurt Shake (Table 1.16, 11)	933	225	28.3	5.2	10.6
40 g ice-cream (dairy)	280	66	10.0	1.4	2.6
Total =	5489	1322	186.5	32.0	52.8
2 5- to 6-year-old					
As above	5489	1322	186.5	32.0	52.8
Plus					
Tomato and Baked Bean Soup (Table 1.16, 12)	500	119	16.2	5.9	3.8
Egg and Orange Juice (Table 1.16, 7)	628	150	19.1	7.1	5.5
25 g glucose polymer	400	100	25.0	—	—
Total =	7017	1691	246.8	45.0	62.1

3 7- to 8-year-old

800 ml milk (whole full fat)	2176	520	37.6	26.4	30.4
80 g glucose polymer	1280	320	80.0	—	—
30 ml Prosparol/Calogen/double cream	555	135	—	—	15
200 ml fruit juice – natural orange juice	323	76	19.0	1.2	—
20 g glucose polymer	335	80	20.0	—	—
Tomato and Baked Bean Soup (Table 1.16, 12)	500	119	16.2	5.9	3.8
Egg and Orange Juice (Table 1.16, 7)	628	150	19.1	7.1	5.5
Yoghurt Shake (Table 1.16, 11)	933	225	28.3	5.2	10.6
Banana Milk Shake (Table 1.16, 9)	929	222	26.5	6.3	10.8
100 g custard	≈ 420	100	14.0	3.3	3.8
Total =	8079	1947	260.7	55.4	79.9

4 9- to 11-year-old

As above	8079	1947	260.7	55.4	79.9
Plus					
1 to 2 drinks Ice-Cream Coke (Table 1.16, 10)	530 to 1060	124 to 248	25.4 to 50.8	1.4 to 2.8	2.6 to 5.2
Total =	8609 to 9139	2071 to 2195	286.1 to 311.5	56.8 to 58.2	82.5 to 85.1

Vitamin mineral supplements are recommended with these regimens, e.g., 6 Cow & Gate Vitamin-Mineral Supplement Tablets (crushed) plus 5 ml Ketovite (Paines & Byrne) liquid. Recommended intakes for different aged children given in **Table 1.2.**

volumes of total feed or in those in whom the feed is poorly tolerated as a bolus feed regimen. It is essential that the position of the nasogastric tube (by aspirate or air) is checked before each bolus feed and at least 4-hourly with continuous enteral feeding. This will also determine whether gastric emptying is occurring.

A gastrostomy is occasionally necessary, for example in patients with oesophageal stricture. As the tubes used are much wider than nasogastric ones, thicker feeds and a wider variety of purée foods can be given.

Jejunostomy or nasojejunum feeding is less desirable as a bolus regimen is not tolerated well; both dumping syndrome, especially with higher osmolar feeds, and steatorrhoea can occur due to inadequate mixing of the feed with bile and pancreatic juice. A predigested feed, e.g., Pregestimil, and/or Flexical (Mead Johnson) can be used to overcome the latter problem and a continuous feeding regimen is recommended.

A variety of nasogastric feed delivery equipment is available for adults which can be adapted and paediatric equipment is becoming available from Viomedex Ltd. (Gordon Rd, Buxted). Gravity drip feeding is not recommended for paediatric patients in whom fluid overload can be a serious hazard. This can be overcome by the use of enteric paediatric feeding pumps or syringe pumps as appropriate for the age and size of the patient and feed volume to be administered. Giving sets should contain a burette for safety to prevent overload of fluid from the reservoir should the clips fail to retain the fluid adequately. The new 'piggy back' battery-operated portable pumps by Viomedex give ambulatory patients more freedom. Nasogastric enteral feeds must be carefully identified so that they are not mistakenly given into a vein. We have found a red-on-white sticker to identify these feeds is useful; it is over-printed 'Nasogastric tube feed, oral use only'. Reverse leur fittings on enteral feed equipment, compared to intravenous equipment, is now becoming standard.

Recipes for home-made basic feeds are given in Table 1.18 and are suitable for the toddler and those for the older child are shown in Table 1.19, and can easily be adjusted for the patient's nutritional requirements. The home-made feeds are considerably lower in cost than commercial preparations. They can be adjusted for individual requirements and should be supplemented with vitamins and trace elements, particularly iron, folic acid and vitamins D and C. They are nutritionally adequate at least for short-term use in the majority of paediatric patients requiring

Table 1.18 Example of enteral feeds for young children (1 to 3 years).

1000 ml	Calcium mmol	Phosphorus mmol	Potassium mmol	Sodium mmol	Energy kJ	Energy kcal	CHO g	Protein g	Fat g
1 1000 ml Milumil (Milupa)	18	17.7	22	12.0	2860	680	84	19.0	31.0
+ 30 g glucose polymer	—	—	—	—	480	120	30	—	—
Total =	18	17.7	22	12.0	3340	800	114	19.0	31.0
2 375 ml (1 can) Clinifeed Iso (Roussel)	5.6	5.2	9.6	5.7	1575	375	49	10.5	15.4
+ 625 ml Milumil (Milupa)	11.3	11.1	13.8	7.5	1788	425	53	11.9	19.4
Total =	16.9	16.3	23.4	13.2	3363	800	102	22.4	34.8
3 750 ml (2 cans) Clinifeed Iso (Roussel)	11.3	10.3	19.2	11.4	3150	750	98	23.0	30.8
250 ml Milumil (Milupa)	4.5	4.5	5.5	3.0	715	170	21	4.8	7.8
Total =	15.8	14.8	24.7	14.4	3865	920	119	27.8	38.6
4 1000 ml Clinifeed Iso (Roussel)	15.2	13.8	25.6	15.2	4200	1000	130	28.0	41.0

An appropriate volume to cover energy needs of the particular patient should be selected from the most suitable feed for the nutritional needs. Vitamin supplements should be given with at least **3** and **4**.

Table 1.19 Example of an enteral feed based on cow's milk for children over 2 years.

	Energy		CHO	Protein	Fat
	kJ	kcal	g	g	g
900 ml milk (full fat homogenized)	2448	585	42.3	29.7	34.2
60 g glucose polymer	960	240	60	—	—
30 ml Prosparol/Calogen/double cream	555	135	—	0 to trace	15
Water to 1000 ml	—	—	—	—	—
Total	3963	960	102.3	29.7	49.2

Vitamin mineral supplements are recommended with this feed including iron and folic acid, e.g. 6 Cow & Gate Vitamin-Mineral Supplement Tablets crushed plus 5 ml Ketovite (Paines & Byrne) liquid **or** 1 Foreceval Junior Capsule (Unigreg) per day (the content only can be given if necessary) **or** Abidec (Parke Davis) 0.6 ml may suffice when the feed is used temporarily.

enteral tube feeding. The feeds should be made with homogenized milk and a suitable oil emulsion in order to ensure adequate fat dispersion to prevent loss of important energy from fat clinging to feed dispensing equipment and tube feed reservoirs.

A variety of commercially available chemically defined enteral feeds (Table 1.20) designed for adult nutrition can be adapted for use in older children. They are not suitable for infants or as the sole source of nutrition in the young child under 5 years. Most are based on cow's milk protein. Lactose is usually well tolerated by children though lactose-free formulae are available. MCT fat is not necessary or desirable for routine fluid diets, and therefore feeds containing MCT should be reserved for patients with steatorrhoea.

Feeds based on hydrolyzates or amino acids are useful for those patients who are either intolerant to cow's milk protein or are fed by jejunostomy or have compromised absorption. They are unpalatable, expensive and have high osmolalities. They are frequently referred to as elemental diets.

A comparison between Clinifeed Iso (Roussel) and normal recommended intakes for different age groups is given (Table 1.21).

Feed Introduction in the Severely Ill Child
Gastric emptying must be established before a fine bore tube can be used or a continuous feeding regimen established. It is difficult to aspirate any fluid through a fine bore tube and therefore at least initially a Ryle's or Portex tube is preferable. The feed is introduced

grading from 5% dextrose or a glucose electrolyte mixture to $\frac{1}{4}$, $\frac{1}{2}$, then full strength feed over several hours or days as clinically appropriate. Slow increase of volume and concentration of feed is important when introducing feeds to a rested gut, or when absorption is compromised or the feed has a high osmolality. However, for the majority a full strength feed can be given immediately and has nutritional advantages (Keohane *et al*. 1984). The technique of tube feeding is described by Grant & Todd (1982).

Fluid diets must be prepared and stored with care as they are easily contaminated and a good media for microbial growth. They should be freshly prepared or stored in a refrigerator for no longer than 24 hours. Liquidizers used in their preparation should be thoroughly washed, dried and sterilized or scalded before each use. Nasogastric and enteral feeds should be prepared under the same rigorous aseptic preparation as infant feeds including terminal pasteurization if a sterile commercial product is not selected. The reservoir of feed should be changed every 4 hours and the giving sets each 24 hours to reduce the risk of microbial contamination.

Diarrhoea in patients who are being fed enteral feeds should be investigated and the following considered:

1. Intercurrent infection in the patient
2. Antibiotic therapy
3. Microbial contamination of feeds and/or equipment
4. Osmolality of the feed and correct dilution of ingredients
5. Delivery time of the feed, i.e., a slower delivery enhances feed tolerance. Small frequent feeding regimen, e.g., 2-hourly × 12 or continuous feed with pump delivery
6. Clinical lactose intolerance which is actually quite rare and an over-rated cause of diarrhoea in the past

Patients who are immobile for long periods are at greater risk of renal calculi. The lower calcium feeds may be preferable in this situation.

Constipation, although not usually a problem with fluid diets, when it does occur, can be corrected by reverting to bolus feeds or administering continuous feeds for only 20 hours maximum per day to encourage peristalsis and so make use of the natural physiological rhythm of fasting, food, and defaecation. Brown sugar in place of part of the feed carbohydrate, the provision of fresh natural orange juice once- or twice-daily, or a small quantity of prune juice will also help relieve constipation. Methyl cellulose

Table 1.20 Adult enteral feeds composition/1000 ml. (Data from manufacturers 1984).

	Clinifeed Iso Vanilla (Roussel)[a]	Clinifeed Select (Roussel)	Ensure (Abbott)	Ensure Plus (Abbott)	Enteral 400 (SHS)	Flexical[d] (Mead Johnson)	Isocal (Mead Johnson)[a]	Nutranel[d] (Roussel)
Dilution per 1000 ml	r.t.f.[e]	2 cans	r.t.f.[g]	r.t.f.	215 g	227 g	r.t.f.	253 g
Protein g	28	50	37	55	29	23[d]	34	40[d]
Energy kJ	4200	4200	4400	6000	4200	4200	4450	4200
kcal	1000	1000	1060	1450	1000	1000	1060	1000
CHO g	130	138[b]	146[b]	200[b]	144[b]	153[b]	133[b]	188[b]
Fat g	41	30	37	53	39[c]	34[c]	44[c]	10[c]
% Energy from protein	11	20	14.2	15.2	11.6	9	13	16
Sodium mmol	15.2	14	37	47.8	27	15.2	23	20.2
Potassium mmol	25.6	28.8	40	48.7	30	32.1	33	36
Calcium mmol	15.2	6.8	13.8	15	11.7	15	15.8	11.6
Phosphorus mmol	13.8	16.9	17.7	19.4	16.1	16.1	17	11.8
Iron mmol	0.13	0.13	0.17	0.26	0.19	0.16	0.17	0.18
Copper μmol	15.7	6.6	17.3	25.2	15.7	15.7	17.3	15.7
Zinc mmol	0.14	0.11	0.24	0.36	0.16	0.15	0.16	0.1
Vitamin A μg	450	494	800	800	813	750	791	750
D μg	4.3	5.0	5.3	5.3	4.8	5.0	5.3	5.0
C mg	40	72	160	159	70.8	150	158	55
Vitamin B_{12} μg	2.5	10	6.4	9.5	4.8	7.5	7.9	2.0
Folic acid μg	140	300	210	211	208	200	211	250
Osmolality mmol/kg	270	387	380	460	300	550	300	410

Dilution per 1000 ml	Nutrauxil (Kabivitrum) r.t.f.	Portagen (Mead Johnson) 200 g[h]	Prosobee (Mead Johnson) 200 g[h]	Complan Natural (Farley) 200 g	Triosorbon (Merck) 212.5 g	Fortison Standard & Soya (Cow & Gate)[a] r.t.f.	Pregestimil[d] (Mead Johnson) 148 g	Comparison with cow's milk Liquid
Protein g	38	33	31.2	40	40.4	40	18.9[d]	33
Energy kJ	4200	3900	4368	3740	4250	4200	2871	2720
kcal	1000	928	1040	888	1000	1000	684	650
CHO g	138[b]	109[b]	103[b]	110	119[b]	120[b]	91.2[b]	47
Fat g	34[c]	45[c]	56	32	40.4[c]	40	27.1[c]	38
% Energy from protein	15	14.2	12	18	16	16	11	20
Sodium mmol	33	19	17	30.4	45	35	13.8	22
Potassium mmol	32	30	23.8	43.6	45	38	18.9	38
Calcium mmol	12.5	22	23.3	36.5	12.5	12.5	15.8	30
Phosphorus mmol	19.4	21.4	20	37.4	19.4	16.1	13.7	30.6
Iron mmol	0.18	0.32	0.33	0.25	0.16	0.18	0.23	0.01
Copper μmol	15.7	23.6	14.2	15.7	15.7	15.7	9.4	3.1
Zinc mmol	0.11	0.13	0.12	0.07	0.11	0.1	0.06	0.05
Vitamin A μg	600	2200	780	700	500	700	633	386
D μg	5.0	18.4	16.2	2.8	5	5.0	10.6	0.4
C mg	50	73.6	84	20	50	50.0	54.9	15
Vitamin B$_{12}$ μg	3	5.9	3.1	4.4	1.5	2	2.1	3
Folic acid μg	200	147	156	110	200	250	106.5	30
Osmolality mmol/kg	350	311	N/s	420	288	300	338	288

All products contain a comprehensive range of other vitamins and minerals. Except for Prosobee (Mead Johnson), Portagen (Mead Johnson) and Pregestimil (Mead Johnson) these products are unsuitable for infants and as the sole source of nutrition in young children under about 5 years old. Other infant feeds are listed in Table 1.6 and modification for toddlers on Table 1.17.

[a] Other products in the range are available including a high energy feed.   [b] Low Lactose Formula.   [c] Partial MCT replacement of fat.   [d] Hydrolysed protein. This type of product is frequently referred to as an elemental diet. Other formulae in this range of products are being developed including some for paediatric patients (see Table 1.6).   [e] Ready-to-feed.   [f] N/s not specified.   [g] Powder 235 g per 1000 ml.   [h] Higher concentration than normal dilution.

Table 1.21 Comparison of one enteral feed with nutritional recommended daily allowance[a] for different ages (girls and boys).

Clinifeed Iso (Roussel)	1-year-old 1000 ml	3- to 4-year-old 1200 ml	5- to 6-year-old 1500 ml	7- to 8-year-old 1750 ml	9- to 11-year-old 2000 ml
Protein g	28 (27–30)	33.6 (37–39)	42 (42–43)	49 (47–49)	56 (51–57)
Energy[c] kcal	1000	1200	1500	1750	2000
kJ	4200	5040	6300	7350	8200
kcal	(1100–1200)	(1500–1560)	(1680–1740)	(1900–1980)	(2050–2280)
% Energy from protein	11.2 (10)	11.2 (10)	11.2 (10)	11.2 (10)	11.2 (10)
Calcium mmol	15 (15[d] 20[e])	18 (15)	22.5 (15)	26.3 (15)	30 (17.5[d] 30[e])
Phosphorus mmol	13.5 (25.8[e])	16.3 (25.8[e])	20.4 (25.8[e])	23.8 (25.8[e])	27 (38.7[e])
Iron mmol	0.13 (0.13)	0.15 (0.14)	0.19 (0.18)	0.22 (0.18)	0.32 (0.22)
Zinc mmol	0.14 (0.15[e])	0.2 (0.15[e])	0.21 (0.15[e])	0.24 (0.15[e])	0.28 (0.23[e])

Vitamin A μg	450 (300)	540 (300)	675 (300)	787.5 (400)	900 (575)
Vitamin B_2 μg	1.2 (0.6)	1.4 (0.8)	1.8 (0.9)	2.1 (1.0)	2.4 (1.2)
Vitamin D[b] μg	4.3 (10)	5.1 (10)	6.4 (10[b])	7.5 (10[b])	8.6 (10[b])
Vitamin B_{12} μg	2.5 (0.9[e])	3.0 (0.9)	3.8 (1.5)	4.4 (1.5)	5 (2[e])
Folic acid μg	140 (100)	166.4 (100)	208 (200)	242.7 (200)	280 (300–200)

[a] Recommended intakes from Table 1.2
[b] No dietary sources may be necessary in older children if the child is sufficiently exposed to sunlight. Supplements should be given to young children
[c] Extra fluid and energy can be provided by fruit juice ± small quantities of glucose polymer supplement
[d] DHSS (1985)
[e] National Research Council (1980)

as Colagel (Eli Lilly) can be added to the feed or given medicinally.
Alternatively lactulose can be prescribed.

PARENTERAL NUTRITION

Patients in whom oral nutrition is not possible should be given
parenteral nutrition. This is both invasive and unphysiological but
can be life-saving in patients with multiple malabsorption, for
example, post gut resection, in whom there is no acceptable
alternative. Optimal nutritional status and growth can be achieved
irrespective of oral intake. Our standard regimen for infants under
10 kg requiring parenteral nutrition is largely based on that
described by Booth & Harries (1982). An excellent chapter on
paediatric nutrition for the older child, including requirements, is
given by Grotte *et al.* (1982) and adult parenteral nutrition is dealt
with by Grant & Todd (1982). Some food or feed via the oral route is
important to maintain oral habits particularly in the infant and
young child and also to prevent atrophic enteropathy, pancreatic
and liver changes associated with total parenteral nutrition (Booth
& Harries 1982). It is our practice to give patients on parenteral
nutrition a small oral intake, e.g., 5 ml, 3-hourly × 8, as this is
preferable to no oral intake even though of negligible nutritional
value.

CHRONIC ILLNESS

The chronically ill and handicapped child should be provided
with an adequate diet in an acceptable form. Feeding may be
time-consuming and the technique may require instruction for
specific handicaps, for example, for children with cleft palate or
spasticity. An excellent booklet *Feeding can be Fun* (Ryan 1975),
published by the Spastic Soceity gives practical advice for feeding
the latter group of children. Where possible the feeding should
progress through the normal changes, from feeds to purée to
mashed, then diced or chopped food, then self-feeding, but these
stages may take months or even years to achieve. In the older child
with progressive neurological disease, previous progress may
regress and feeding must be appropriate for the child's condition.

Adequate nutritional intake for growth is essential. Malnutrition
and dental caries which further inhibit adequate intake are
common in this group of patients. Oral hygiene and prevention of

dental caries is important as the latter causes pain and results in further reluctance with eating. A purée or fluid diet (Tables 1.17 to 1.21) may be required in some children with handicap. A wide variety of foods can be puréed in an electric blender/liquidizer, most foods coming from the family meals. Whole full-fat milk is an important basis of such diets and can be used as the fluid needed to purée foods so avoiding low energy concentration to volume which is a common problem with such diets. Most soups are too low in protein and energy value for meal replacement, but are a useful basis in which to liquidize meat and vegetable dishes, so providing a variety of tastes and minerals. A general vitamin supplement is recommended, e.g., 0.6 ml Abidec (Parke Davis).

Obesity may also occur, for example, in the over-indulged child with a handicap in whom energy expenditure is limited, such as those with spina bifada (see Chapter 2).

USEFUL ADDRESSES

Association of Breastfeeding Mothers, 71 Hall Drive, London SE26 6XL

Breastfeeding Promotion Group, National Childbirth Trust, 9 Queensborough Terrace, Bayswater, London W2 3TB

Commission for Racial Equality, Elliot House, 10/12 Allington Street, London SW1E 5EH

The Islamic Foundation, 223 London Road, Leicester LE2 1ZE

Jewish Memorial Council, Woburn House, Upper Woburn Place, London WC1

The King Edwards Hospital Fund for London, 126 Albert Street, London NW1 7NF

La Leche League of Great Britain, PO Box BM 3424, London WC1

London Board of Shecita, Administrative Offices, 1 Bridge Lane, Temple Fortune, Finchley Road, London NW11 0EA

Office of the Chief Rabbi, Adler House, Tavistock Square, London WC1

The Spastics Society, 12 Park Crescent, London W1

The Supreme Council of Sikhs, 162 Great West Road, Hounslow, Middlesex

The Vegan Society, 47 Highlands Road, Leatherhead, Surrey

The Vegetarian Society, 53 Marloes Road, Kensington, London W8 6LA

RECOMMENDED READING FOR COMPOSING
CULTURAL DIETS

CAMERON M. & HOFVANDER Y. (1983) *Manual on Feeding Infants and Young Children*, 3rd ed. Oxford University Press, Oxford.

COMMISSION FOR RACIAL EQUALITY (1977) *A Guide to Asian Diets*. Commission for Racial Equality, London.

DHSS (1981b) *Health Service Catering Manual. Volume 6: Catering for Minority Groups*. HMSO, London.

JEWISH MEMORIAL COUNCIL (1972) *The Practical Guide to Kashrut, Wagschal*. Jewish Memorial Council, London.

MCDERMOTT M. Y. (1980) *The Muslim Guide for Teachers, Employers, Community Workers and Social Administrators in Britain*. The Islamic Foundation, Leicester.

REFERENCES

ADACHI S. & PATTON S. (1961) Presence and significance of lactulose in milk products: a review. *Journal of Dairy Science* **44**, 1375–93.

AGGETT P. J. & DAVIES N. N. (1983) Some nutritional aspects of trace metals. *Journal of Inherited Metabolic Disease* **6**, 22–30.

AHN C. & MACLEAN W. C. (1980) Growth of the exclusively breastfed infant. *American Journal of Clinical Nutrition* **33**, 183–92.

AHRENS E. H. (1979) Dietary fats and coronary heart disease: unfinished business. *Lancet* **2**, 1345–48.

AMERICAN ACADEMY OF PEDIATRICS COMMITTEE ON NUTRITION (1976) Commentary on breast feeding and infant formulae, including proposed standards for formulae. *Pediatrics* **57**, 278.

AMERICAN ACADEMY OF PEDIATRICS COMMITTEE ON NUTRITION (1977) Nutritional needs of low birth-weight infants. *Pediatrics* **60**, 519.

ANDERSSON H., NÄVERT B., BINGHAM S. A., ENGLYST H. N. & CUMMINGS J. H. (1983) The effects of bread containing similar amounts of phytate but different amounts of wheat bran on calcium, zinc and iron balance in man. *British Journal of Nutrition* **50**, 503–10.

ASHKENAZI A., LEVIN S., DJALDETTI M., FISHAL E. & BENVENISH D. (1973) The syndrome of neonatal copper deficiency. *Pediatrics* **53**, 525–33.

ATKINSON S. A., BRYAN M. H. & ANDERSON G. H. (1978) Human milk: differences in nitrogen concentration in milk from mothers of term and preterm infants. *Journal of Pediatrics* **93**, 67.

ATKINSON S. A., RADDE I. C., CHANCE G. W., BRYAN M. H. & ANDERSON G. H. (1980) Macro-mineral content of milk obtained during early lactation from mothers of premature infants. *Early Human Development* **4**, 5–14.

BARLOW B., SANTULLI T. V., HEIRD W. C., PITT J., BLANC W. A. & SCHULLINGER

J. N. (1974) An experimental study of acute neonatal enterocolitis: the importance of breast milk. *Journal of Pediatric Surgery* **9**, 587–94.

BARLTROP D. (1974) Lipid composition and absorption by low birthweight infants. *Pediatric Research* **8**, 138.

BENTOVIM A. (1970) The clinical approach to feeding disorders of childhood. *Journal of Psychosomatic Research* **14**, 267.

BLUMENTHAL I., LEALMAN G. T. & SHOESMITH D. R. (1980) Effect of feed temperature and phototherapy on gastric emptying in the neonate. *Archives of Disease in Childhood* **55**, 562–4.

BOOTH I. & HARRIES J. T. (1982) Parenteral nutrition in young children. *British Journal of Intravenous Therapy* **3**, 31–40.

BOOTH I. W., LEVINE M. M. & HARRIES J. T. (1984) Oral rehydration therapy in acute diarrhoea in childhood. *Journal of Paediatrics* **3**, 491–9.

BROOKE O. G., WOOD C. & BAILEY J. (1982) Energy balance, nitrogen balance and growth in preterm infants fed expressed breast milk, a premature infant formula, and two low solute formulae. *Archives of Disease in Childhood* **57**, 898–904.

BUNKER V. W. & CLAYTON B. E. (1983) Trace element content of commercial enteral feeds. *Lancet* **2**, 426–8.

BURKITT D., MORLEY D. & WALKER A. (1980) Dietary fibre in under and over nutrition. *Archives of Disease in Childhood* **55**, 803–7.

BURMAN D. (1982) Nutrition in early childhood. In McLaren D. S. & Burman D. (eds) *Textbook of Paediatric Nutrition*, 2nd ed., pp.39–73. Churchill Livingstone, Edinburgh.

BUTLER A. M. & RICHIE R. N. (1960) Simplification and improvement in estimating drug dosage, fluid and dietary allowance for patients of varying sizes. *New England Journal of Medicine* **262**, 903.

CAMERON M. & HOFVANDER Y. (1983) *Manual on Feeding Infants and Young Children*, 3rd ed. Oxford University Press, Oxford.

CATZEL P. (1974) *The Paediatric Prescriber*, 4th ed., p.7. Blackwell Scientific Publications, Oxford.

CHANDRA R. K. (1981) Breastfeeding, growth and morbidity. *Nutrition Research* **1**, 25–31.

CHETLEY A. (1979) *The Baby Killer Scandal*. Published by War on Want, London.

COMMISSION FOR RACIAL EQUALITY (1977) *A Guide to Asian Diets*. Commission for Racial Equality, London.

CRAWFORD M. A., HASSAM A. G., WILLIAMS G. & WHITEHOUSE W. L. (1976) Essential fatty acids and fetal brain growth. *Lancet* **1**, 452.

CRISP, A. H. (1977) Anorexia nervosa. *Proceedings of the Royal Society of Medicine* **70**, 464 & 686. William Clowes & Sons Ltd, London.

CUTHBERTSON D. P. (1980) Alterations in metabolism following injury. *Injury* **2**, 175–89 & 286–303.

DAVIES D. P. (1977) Adequacy of expressed breast milk for early growth in preterm infants. *Archives of Disease in Childhood* **52**, 296–301.

DAVIES D. P. (1979) Is inadequate breastfeeding an important cause of failure to thrive? *Lancet* **1**, 541.

DAVIES P. A. & RUSSELL H. (1968) Later progress of 100 infants weighing 1000 to 2000g at birth fed immediately with breast milk. *Developmental Medicine and Child Neurology* **10**, 725.

DeCARVALHO M., ROBERTSON S., FRIEDMAN A. & KLAUS M. (1983) Effect of frequent breastfeeding on early milk production and infant weight gain. *Pediatrics* **72**, 307–11.

DHSS (1977) *The Composition of Mature Human Milk.* Report No. 12. HMSO, London.

DHSS (1980a) *Artificial Feeds for the Young Infant.* Report No. 18. HMSO, London.

DHSS (1980b) *Rickets and Osteomalacia.* Report No. 19. HMSO, London.

DHSS (1981a) *The Collection and Storage of Human Milk.* Report No. 22. HMSO, London.

DHSS (1981b) *Health Service Catering Manual, Vol. 6. Catering for Minority Groups.* HMSO, London.

DHSS (1983, revised) *Present Day Practice in Infant Feeding.* Report No. 20. (1980) HMSO, London.

DHSS (1984) *Diet and Cardiovascular Disease.* Report No. 28. HMSO, London.

DHSS (1985, revised) *Recommended Daily Amounts of Food Energy and Nutrients for Groups of People in the United Kingdom.* Report No. 15. (1979) HMSO, London.

DOBBING J. & SANDS J. (1973) The quantitive growth and development of the human brain. *Archives of Disease in Childhood* **48**, 757–67.

DOBBING J. (1974) Later development of the brain and its vulnerability. In Davis J. A. & Dobbing J. (eds) *Scientific Foundations of Paediatrics,* p.565. Heinemann Medical, London.

Drug and Therapeutics Bulletin, Editorial (1983) Cow's milk substitutes. *Drug and Therapeutics Bulletin* **21**, 94–6.

EBRAHIM G. J. (1978) *Breastfeeding: The Biological Option.* Macmillan, London.

ELWYN D. H. (1980) Nutritional requirements of adult surgical patients. *Critical Care Medicine* **8**, 9–20.

EYAL F., SAGI E., ARAD I. & AVITAL A. (1982) Necrotising enterocolitis in the very low birthweight infant: expressed breast milk compared with parenteral feeding. *Archives of Disease in Childhood* **57**, 274–6.

FAO/WHO (1970) *Nutritional Studies: Amino Acid Content of Foods and Biological Data on Proteins,* No. 24, p.134. FAO, Rome.

FAO/WHO (1973) *Energy and Protein Requirements.* Report of a joint FAO/WHO ad-hoc expert committee (WHO Technical Report Series No. 522 and FAO Nutrition Meetings Report Series No. 52, Geneva.

FAO/WHO (1975) *Energy and Protein Requirements.* Recommendations by a joint FAO/WHO informal gathering of experts. *Food and Nutrition* **1**, 11–19.

FAO/WHO (1976) Recommended International Standards for Foods for Infants and Children. Joint FAO/WHO Food Standards Programme. Codex Alimentarius Commission. FAO, Rome.

FAO/WHO (1978) An Examination of Current Recommendations on Requirements for Protein and Energy. Report of consultants meeting in Rome, 15th–17th October, 1977. FAO, Rome.

FAO/WHO (1980) Dietary Fats and Oils in Human Nutrition. FAO of the United Nations, pp.21–37. FAO, Rome.

FERGUSSON D. M., HORWOOD, L. J., BEAUTRAIS A. L., SHANNON F. T. & TAYLOR B. (1981) Eczema and infant diet. Clinical Allergy 11, 325–31.

FOMAN S. J., ZIEGLER E. E., THOMAS L. N., JENSEN R. L. & FILER L. J. (1970) Excretion of fat by normal full-term infants fed various milks and formulas. American Journal of Clinical Nutrition 23, 1299–1313.

FRANCIS D. E. M. (1984a) The infant feeding controversy. Nursing 22, 635–8.

FRANCIS D. E. M. (1984b) Should we be advising low fat diets in the United Kingdom? Health Visitor 57, 145–6.

FRANCIS, D. E. M. (1985) Food, fats and facts for nutrition in children. Nursing 39, 1149–52.

FRANCIS D. E. M. (in press) Diets for Sick Children, 4th edn. Blackwell Scientific Publications, Oxford.

GAULL G. E., RASSIN, D. K., RÄIHÄ N. C. R. & HEINONEN K. (1977) Milk protein quantity and quality in low birthweight infants, III. Effect of sulphur amino acids in plasma and urine. Journal of Pediatrics 90, 348–55.

GIBBS J. H., FISHER C., BHATTACHARYA S., GODDARD P. & BAUM J. D. (1977) Drip breast milk; its composition, collection and pasteurization. Early Human Development 1, 227–45.

GLASER J. & JOHNSTONE D. E. (1953) Prophylaxis of allergic disease in newborn. Journal of the American Medical Association 153, 620–22.

GOLDMAN H. I., GOLDMAN S., KAUFMAN I. R. & LIEBMAN O. B. (1974) Late effects of early dietary protein intake on low birthweight infants. Journal of Pediatrics 85, 764.

GRANATH L. E., ROOTZEN H., LILJEGREN E. et al. (1976) Variation in caries prevalence related to combinations of dietary and oral hygiene habits in 6-year-old children. Caries Research 10, 308–17.

GRANT A. & TODD E. (1982) Enteral and Parenteral Nutrition. Blackwell Scientific Publications, Oxford.

GROTTE, G., MEURLING S. & WRETLIND A. (1982) Parenteral nutrition. In McLaren D. S. & Burman D. (eds) Textbook of Paediatric Nutrition, 2nd ed., pp.228–58. Churchill Livingstone, Edinburgh.

HANSEN A. E., STEWART, R., HUGHES G. & SÖDERHJELM LARS. (1962) The relation of linoleic acid to infant feeding. A review. Acta Paediatric Scandinavica Supplement 137, 721–6.

HANSEN J. D. L., BUCHANAN N. & PETTIFOR J. M. (1982) Protein energy malnutrition. In McLaren D. S. & Burman D. (eds) Textbook of

Paediatric Nutrition, 2nd ed., pp.114–42. Churchill Livingstone, Edinburgh.

HAROON Y., SHEARER M. J., RAHIM S., GUNN W. G., McENERY G. & BARKHAN P. (1982) The content of phylloquinone (Vitamin K_1) in human milk, cow's milk and infant formula foods determined by high performance liquid chromatography. *The Journal of Nutrition* **112,** 1105–17.

HAWORTH C. & EVANS D. I. K. (1981) Nutritional aspects of blood disorders in the newborn. *Journal of Human Nutrition* **35,** 323–34.

HEIRD W. C., DRISCOLL J. M., SCHULLINGER J. N., GREBIN B. & WINTERS R. W. (1972) Intravenous alimentation in pediatric patients. *Journal of Pediatrics* **8,** 351–72.

HOLMES G. E., HASSANEIN K. M. & MILLER H. C. (1983) Factors associated with infections among breast fed babies and babies fed proprietary milks. *Pediatrics* **72,** 300–6.

HUGHES C., DUTTON S. & TRUSWELL A. S. (1981) High intakes of ascorbic acid and urinary oxalate. *Journal of Human Nutrition* **35,** 274–80.

INFIRRI J. S. (1984) Trends in the pattern of oral disease: Implications for Ireland. *Journal of Irish Dental Association* April–June, 13–19.

JAMES W. P. T. (1981) Protein and energy metabolism after trauma. *Acta Chirurgica Scandinavica* Supplement 507, 1.

JAMES W. P. T. (1983) Proposals for Nutritional Guidelines for Health Education in Britain. A discussion paper. National Advisory Committee on Nutrition Education. Health Education Council, London.

JELLIFFE D. B. & JELLIFFE E. F. (1978) *Human Milk in the Modern World.* Oxford University Press, Oxford.

JIVANI S. K. M. (1978) The practice of infant feeding among Asian immigrants. *Archives of Disease in Childhood* **53,** 69–73.

KEOHANE P. P., ATTRILL H., LOVE M., FROST P. & SILK D. B. A. (1984) Relation between osmolality of diet and gastrointestinal side effects in enteral nutrition. *British Medical Journal* **288,** 678–80.

KOCHHAR S. P. & MATSUI T. (1984) Essential fatty acids and *trans* contents of some oils, margarines and other fats. *Food Chemistry* **13,** 85–101.

LAKDAWALA D. R. & WIDDOWSON E. M. (1977) Vitamin D in human milk. *Lancet* **1,** 167–8.

Lancet, Editorial (1981) Dental caries and fluoride. *Lancet* **1,** 1351.

Lancet, Editorial (1984) Is reduction in blood cholesterol effective? *Lancet* **1,** 317.

LENTER C. (ed.) (1981) Geigy Scientific Tables vol. 1, Units of Measurement, Body Fluids, Composition of the Body, Nutrition, 8th revised ed, pp.213–16. Ciba-Geigy, Basle.

LUCAS A., GIBBS J. A. M. & BAUM J. D. (1978) The biology of human drip breast milk. *Early Human Development* **2,** 351–61.

LUCAS A., LUCAS P. J., CHAVIN S. I., LYSTER R. L. J. & BAUM J. D. (1980) A human milk formula. *Early Human Nutrition* **4,** 15–21.

LUCAS A., GORE S. M., COLE T. J., BAMFORD M. F., DOSSETOR J. F. B., BARR I., DICARLO L., CORK S. & LUCAS P. J. (1984) Multicentre trial on feeding low birthweight infants: effects of diet on early growth. *Archives of Disease in Childhood* **59,** 722–30.

McClelland D. B. L., McGrath J. & Samson R. R. (1978) Antimicrobial factors in human milk. *Acta Pediatrica Scandinavica* Supplement 271, 1–20.

McDermott M. Y. (1980) 'The Muslim Guide' for Teachers, Employers, Community Workers and Social Administrators in Britain. The Islamic Foundation, Leicester.

McKillop F. M. & Durnin J. V. G. A. (1982) The energy and nutritional intake of a random sample (305) of infants. *Human Nutrition, Applied Nutrition* **36A,** 405–21.

McLaren D. S. (1982a) Nutritional assessment. In McLaren D. S. & Burman D. (eds) *Textbook of Paediatric Nutrition,* 2nd ed., pp. 88–99. Churchill Livingstone, Edinburgh.

McLaren D. S. (1982b) Protein energy malnutrition. In McLaren D. S. & Burman D. (eds) *Textbook of Paediatric Nutrition,* 2nd ed., pp.103–13. Churchill Livingstone, Edinburgh.

McLaren D. S. & Burman D. (1982) *Textbook of Paediatric Nutrition,* 2nd ed. Churchill Livingstone, Edinburgh.

McLaughlin P., Anderson K. J., Widdowson E. M. & Coombs R. R. A. (1981) Effect of heat on the anaphylactic sensitising capacity of cow's milk, goat's milk and various infant formulae fed to guinea pigs. *Archives of Disease in Childhood* **56,** 165–71.

McMillan J. A., Landow S. A. & Oski F. A. (1976) Iron sufficiency in breast fed infants and the availability of iron from human milk. *Pediatrics* **58,** 686–91.

Macy I. G. & Kelly J. H. (1961) Human and cow's milk in infant nutrition. In Kon S. K. & Cowie A. T. (eds) *Milk: the mammary gland and its secretion,* Volume II, pp.265–304. Academic Press, New York.

Mamunes P., Prince P. E., Thornton N., Hunt P. A. & Hitchcock, E. S. (1976) Intellectual deficits after transient tyrosinaemia in the term neonate. *Pediatrics* **57,** 675–80.

Magarey A. & Boulton J. C. (1984) Nutritional studies during childhood: IV Energy and nutrient intake at age 4. *Australian Paediatric Journal* **20,** 187–94.

Martin D. J. & Monk J. (1982) *Infant Feeding 1980.* Office of Population Censuses and Surveys, St. Catherine's House, 10 Kingsway, London WC2 6JP.

Matthew D. J., Taylor B., Norman A. P., Turner M. W. & Soothill J. F. (1977) Prevention of eczema. *Lancet* **1,** 321–7.

Mendelson R. A., Bryan M. H. & Anderson G. H. (1983) Trace mineral balances in preterm infants fed their own mother's milk. *Journal of Pediatric Gastroenterology and Nutrition* **2,** 256–61.

Mendez A. & Olano A. (1979) Lactulose. A review of some chemical properties and applications in infant nutrition and medicine. *Dairy Science Abstracts* **41,** 531–5.

Menkes J. H., Welcher D. W., Levi H.S., Dallas J. & Gretsky N. E. (1972)

Relationship of elevated blood tyrosine to the ultimate intellectual performance of premature infants. *Pediatrics* **49**, 218–24.

METCOFF J. (1982) Maternal nutrition and fetal growth. In McLaren D. S. & Burman D. (eds) *Textbook of Paediatric Nutrition*, 2nd ed., pp.18–38. Churchill Livingstone, Edinburgh.

MITCHELL J. R. A. (1984) What constitutes evidence on the dietary prevention of coronary heart disease? Cosy beliefs or harsh facts? *International Journal of Cardiology* **5**, 287–98.

MOORE T. (1984) Food advice goes into reverse: 1983 vs 1936. Personal views with a long look back. *Human Nutrition: Applied Nutrition* **38A**, 337–44.

MUNRO H. N. (1979) Hormones and the metabolic response to injury. *New England Journal of Medicine* **300**, 41.

NAISMITH D. J., DEEPROSE S. P., SUPRAMANIAM G. & WILLIAMS M. J. H. (1978) Reappraisal of linoleic acid requirement of the young infant with particular regard to use of modified cow's milk. *Archives of Disease in Childhood* **53**, 845–9.

NARAYANAN I., PRAKASH K., PRABHAKAR A. K. & GUJRAL V. V. (1982a) A planned prospective evaluation of the anti-infective property of varying quantities of expressed human milk. *Acta Paediatrica Scandinavica* **71**, 441–5.

NARAYANAN I., PRAKASH K. & GUJRAL V. V. (1982b) Management of expressed human milk in a developing country—experiences and practical guidelines. *Journal of Tropical Paediatrics* **28**, 25–7.

NARAYANAN I., SINGH B. & HARVEY D. (1984) Fat loss during feeding of human milk. *Archives of Disease in Childhood* **59**, 475–7.

NATIONAL RESEARCH COUNCIL (1980) *Food and Nutrition Board Recommended Dietary Allowances*, 9th revised edn. National Academy of Sciences, Washington DC.

NELIGAN G. A., KOLVIN I., SCOTT D. & GARSIDE R. F. (1976) Born too soon or born too small. *Clinics in Developmental Medicine* No. 61. Heinemann Medical, London.

NORTON K. (1983) Anorexia nervosa. *Midwife, Health Visitor and Community Nurse* **19**, 310–14.

OLIVER M. F. (1984) Hypercholesterolaemia and coronary heart disease: an answer. *British Medical Journal* **288**, 423.

OUNSTED M. & SLEIGH G. (1975) The infant's self regulation of food intake and weight gain. *Lancet* **1**, 1393–7.

PASSMORE R., HOLLINGSWORTH D. F. & ROBERTSON J. (1979) Prescription for a better British diet. *British Medical Journal* **1**, 527–31.

PAUL A. A. & SOUTHGATE D. A. T. (1978) *McCance & Widdowson's The Composition of Foods*, 4th ed. HMSO, London.

POHLANDT F. (1974) Cystine: a semi-essential amino acid in the newborn infant. *Acta Paediatrica Scandinavica* **63**, 801.

PUGH P. J. (1982) Neonatal hypoglycaemia: notes and queries. *Practitioner* **226**, 385.

RAIHA N. C., HEINONEN K. & RASSIN D. K. (1976) Milk protein quantity and quality in low birthweight infants. I. Metabolic response and effects on growth. *Paediatrics* **57,** 659–84.

RASSIN D. K., GAULL G. E., RAIHA N. C. R. & HEINONEN K. (1977) Milk protein quantity and quality in low birthweight infants. *Journal of Pediatrics* **90,** 356–60.

RATTIGAN S., GHISALBERTI A. V. & HARTMAN P. E. (1981) Breast milk production in Australian women. *British Journal of Nutrition* **45,** 243–9.

RICHARDS J. R. (1977) Metabolic reponse to injury, infection and starvation, an overview. In Richards J. R. & Kinney J. M. (eds) *Nutritional Aspects of Care in the Critically Ill*, p.273. Churchill Livingstone, Edinburgh.

ROBERTS I. F., WEST R. J., OGILVIE D. & DILLON M. (1979) Malnutrition in infants receiving cult diets: a cause of child abuse. *British Medical Journal* **1,** 296–8.

ROY R. N., CHANCE G. W., RADDE I. C., HILL D. E., WILLIS D. M. & SHEEPERS, J. (1976) Late hyponatraemia in very low birthweight infants (>1.3 kg). *Pediatric Research* **10,** 526–31.

RYAN M. (1975) *Feeding Can be Fun: Advice on Feeding Handicapped Babies and Children*. Published by the Spastic Society, Meadway Works, Birmingham.

SAARINEN U. M., KAJOSAARI M., BACKMAN A. & SIIMES M. A. (1979) Prolonged breastfeeding as prophylaxis for atopic disease. *Lancet* **2,** 163–8.

SAHASHI Y., SUZUKI T., HIGAKI M. & ASANO T. (1967) Metabolism of Vitamin D in animals, 5. Isolation of Vitamin D sulphate from human milk. *Journal of Vitaminology*, Japan, **13,** 33–6.

SMITH I. & FRANCIS D. E. M. (1982) Disorders of amino acid metabolism. In McLaren D. S. & Burman D. (eds) *Textbook of Paediatric Nutrition*, 2nd ed., pp.295–323. Churchill Livingstone, Edinburgh.

SNYDERMAN S. E., HOLT L. E., NORTON P. M., ROITMAN E. & PHANSALKAR S. V. (1968) The plasma aminogram I. Influence of the level of protein intake and a comparison of whole protein and amino acid diets. *Pediatric Research* **2,** 131.

SOOTHILL J. F. (1982) Prevention of food allergy. In Challacombe S. & Brostoff J. (eds) *Clinics in Immunology and Allergy* Vol 2, No. 1, pp.243–55. W. B. Saunders, Eastbourne.

SUTHERLAND A. B. (1976) Nitrogen balance and nutritional requirements in the burn patient; a reappraisal. *Burns* 2, 238–44.

TANNER J. M. & THOMSON A. M. (1970) Standards for birthweight at gestation periods from 32 to 42 weeks allowing for maternal height and weight. *Archives of Disease in Childhood* **45,** 566.

TANNER J. M. & WHITEHOUSE R. H. (1976) Clinical longitudinal standards for height, weight, height velocity, weight velocity and stages of puberty. *Archives of Disease in Childhood* **51,** 170.

THOMAS, L. H., JONES P. R., WINTER J. A. & SMITH H. (1981) Hydrogenated oils and fats: the presence of chemically-modified fatty acids in human adipose tissue. *The American Journal of Clinical Nutrition* **34,** 877–86.

TRIPP J. H., FRANCIS D. E. M., KNIGHT J. A. & HARRIES, J. T. (1979) Infant feeding practices: a cause for concern. *British Medical Journal* **2,** 707–9.

UNDERWOOD E. J. (1977) *Trace Elements in Human and Animal Nutrition,* 4th ed. Academic Press, London.

VAN CAMPEN D. (1974) Regulation of iron absorption. *Federation Proceedings* **33,** 100–5.

WAGSCHAL S. (1972) *The Practical Guide to Kashrut.* Jewish Memorial Council, London.

WHARTON B. A. & BERGER, H. M. (1976) Bottle feeding. *British Medical Journal* **1,** 1326–31.

WHITEHEAD R. G., PAUL A. A. & ROWLAND M. G. M. (1980) Lactation in Cambridge and The Gambia. *British Medical Bulletin* **37,** 77–82.

WHITEHEAD R. G., PAUL A. A. & COLE T. J. (1981) A critical analysis of measured food energy intakes during infancy and early childhood in comparison with current international recommendations. *Journal of Human Nutrition* **35,** 339–48.

WILLIAMS A. F. & BAUM J. D. (1984) (eds) *Human Milk Banking,* Nestlé Nutrition Workshop Series, vol. 8. Raven, New York.

WILLIAMSON S., HEWITT J. H., FINUCANE E. & GAMSU H. R. (1978a) Organisation of bank of raw and pasteurized human milk for neonatal intensive care. *British Medical Journal* **1,** 393–6.

WILLIAMSON S., FINUCANE E., ELLIS H. & GAMSU H. R. (1978b) Effect of heat treatment of human milk on absorption of nitrogen, fat, sodium, calcium and phosphorus by preterm infants. *Archives of Disease in Childhood* **53,** 553–63.

WISE A. (1983) Dietary factors determining the biological activities of phytate. *Nutrition Abstracts and Reviews in Clinical Nutrition,* Series A, **53,** 791–806.

WOODRUFF C. W., WRIGHT S. W. & WRIGHT R. P. (1972) The role of fresh cow's milk in iron deficiency. *American Journal of Diseases of Children* **124,** 26–30.

WOOLFSON A. M. J., RICKETTS C. R., HARDY S. M. *et al.* (1979) Prolonged nasogastric tube feeding in critically ill and surgical patients. *Postgraduate Medical Journal* **52,** 678–82.

WHO (1974) *Handbook on Human Nutritional Requirements.* Monograph series No. 61. WHO, Geneva.

WHO (1978) *A Growth Chart for International Use in Maternal and Child Health Care.* WHO, Geneva.

WHO (1981) *International Code of Marketing of Breast Milk Substitutes.* WHO, Geneva.

WHO (1982) Expert committee. *Prevention of Coronary Heart Disease.* Technical Report Series No. 678. WHO, Geneva.

World Medicine, Editorial (1984) Eat your heart out. *World Medicine*, 21 March.

YEUNG D. L., PENNELL M. D., LEUNG M. & HALL J. (1982) The effect of 2% milk on infant nutrition. *Nutrition Research* **2,** 651–60.

ZIEGLER E. E., BIGA R. L. & FOMON S. J. (1981) *Textbook of Nutritional Requirements of the Preterm Infant.* Raven, New York.

CHAPTER 2

Overweight and Obesity

The recent report by the Royal College of Physicians chaired by Sir Douglas Black (1983) has extensively reviewed the prevalence, health consequences, causes and management of obesity in the UK. Overweight and obesity are conditions in which there is excessive accumulation of adipose fat. They are the result of excess energy intake over expenditure (Garrow 1978).

Obesity has been defined for adults as a weight of 120% or more of the acceptable range for sex and height, representing a body mass index (BMI), i.e. $Wt \div Ht^2$, of 30 kg/m^2 in men and 28.6 kg/m^2 in women. No adjustment is made for age in adults. Overweight is used to define those individuals whose weight exceeds the upper limit of acceptable weight for sex and height with a BMI over 25 kg/m^2 in men and 23.8 kg/m^2 in women. Tables giving acceptable weight ranges are given in the Royal College of Physicians Obesity Report (Black 1983). Confusion regarding the definitions for children of overweight and obesity have occurred in the past. The obesity report suggests that only those children whose weight exceeds the median + 2 standard deviations for age and sex should be considered abnormal and this should be termed *overweight*. This means all children who fall within the full percentile range for the population are normal and only those whose weight is above the 97th percentile for height and age are overweight. Ideally international National Child Health Statistics (NCHS) reference charts should be used rather than data from an individual population. The NCHS data for 2- to 18-year-olds is given in Black (1983). Weight for height and age may be a more appropriate expression of growth and the data based on pre-war USA statistics, when obesity was less common, is also published in the Obesity Report (Black 1983). BMI cannot be used for children and adolescents unless different standard values for p are used at different ages in the equation kg weight $\div$ m height $_p$, as this would assume BMI is unrelated to height which may not be relevant in children.

· Skinfold thickness measurements with calipers are a more

appropriate estimation of total body fat (Brook 1971). A skinfold thickness in at least one site in excess of 20 mm or combined value for the four skinfold thicknesses of 80 mm indicates obesity. In clinical practice a skinfold thickness over 25 mm (1 inch) measured between finger and thumb is a useful quick guide (Craddock 1982).

Overweight and obesity are the commonest nutritional disorders in Britain accounting for 5 to 39% of adults at different ages, though prevalence of figures in different papers vary. In children the prevalence changes with age. It is most common in adolescence: 9.6% girls and 6.5% boys aged 14 years, compared to 2.9% girls and 1.7% boys aged 6 years, are overweight (Stark et al. 1981), i.e. overall approximately 5% children are overweight. An inappropriate weight gain is common in the 20s age group. It is largely associated with our affluent society. Children of overweight parents are particularly at risk of becoming overweight.

Overweight and obesity should be regarded as a potential health hazard. Infants who are overweight have a higher incidence of minor illness such as respiratory infections (Tracey et al. 1971), and many excessively heavy infants have delayed recovery from pneumonia. Overweight can be associated with raised fasting blood sugar levels and increased blood pressure (Abraham et al. 1971). Adult patients who are obese have an increased chance of diabetes compared with the non-obese. Particular care is needed where there is a family history of diabetes to prevent the development of obesity.

Although coronary heart disease (CHD) is multifactorial, there is an increasing risk of mortality from CHD with overweight (Black 1983). Changes in body weight affect two of the risk factors; blood pressure and serum cholesterol, both of which are reduced with weight loss. Those individuals with a family history of diabetes, hypertension and CHD, and those fat in their twenties, are likely to be particularly susceptible to ill health (Black 1983).

The increased prevalence of overweight in infancy seen in the UK in the 1970s appears to be decreasing (DHSS 1983, revised). This change is no doubt due to a number of factors, but is related to a greater awareness of the dangers of overweight, the increased incidence of breast-feeding and correct use of modified infant formulae in bottle-fed infants. It is important that the harmful effects of obesity are not over emphasised. Fat accumulation during the first 9 months of life is normal and is lost with subsequent increased physical activity in the toddler (Brook 1974).

My earlier suggestion (Francis 1974) on long-term prognosis that

80% of overweight children would become overweight adults were based on published studies on the follow-up of treated patients and have not been confirmed in the recent studies or population surveys (Craddock 1982; Poskitt & Cole 1977; Stark *et al.* 1981). The recently published National Survey of Health and Development (Stark *et al.* 1981) provides an analysis of the relationship between childhood and adult weights. The risk of being overweight in adulthood was related to the degree of overweight in childhood but less than half the overweight 7-year-olds became overweight adults. In a previous analysis of UK studies on the prevalence of overweight children (DHSS/MRC 1976) it was evident that about 35% of children were overweight at 1 year old but this fell to 7% by the age of 6 to 11 years. In adolescence a further increase in the proportion of children categorized as overweight was noted. Given a changing prevalence rate of overweight with age it is incorrect to consider infantile or childhood obesity as an inevitable cause of adult obesity (Poskitt & Cole 1977). However, overweight children are more likely to become overweight adults than their non-obese counterparts (Peckham *et al.* 1983; Black 1983). Those who slim down in later childhood also have an increased risk of becoming overweight in adult life. They should therefore be encouraged to develop eating habits and exercise patterns which will prevent inappropriate weight gains. An increased risk does not signify that overfeeding in infancy was responsible; excess weight at both times may simply reflect the consequences of inappropriate feeding in those predisposed to overweight (Black 1983).

Childhood overweight should not go unchecked (Lloyd 1977). Prevention is, of course, better than cure and the establishment of good food habits from early childhood is of the greatest importance. In seeking to prevent over-nutrition it is important not to produce a swing towards under-nutrition. Chapter 1 gives suggestions regarding normal nutrition which can be adapted for use in preventing and treating overweight. A nutritionally adequate diet can be selected from the food groups (Table 1.11) taking care to avoid or limit the high energy density foods containing large quantities of fats and sugar.

AETIOLOGY

Various genetic and environmental factors contribute to overweight. If both parents are obese they are 8 to 10 times more likely to have children who are overweight than parents of normal weight, and if one parent is overweight the child has 4 times the probability of overweight compared with the child of normal weight parents (Garn & Clark 1976).

GENETIC FACTORS

There is overwhelming and accumulating evidence for a genetic component in overweight, especially in cases of moderate to severe obesity (Craddock 1982) and obesity that persists from infancy (Court & Dunlop 1975). The study of twins has shown monozygous twins have more similar weights and skinfold measurements than heterozygous twins. This and other evidence, summarized by Craddock (1978) and Bray (1981) including studies on adopted children, the fact that fat and lean children can occur in the same family, and family resemblance in regional fat distribution, supports the evidence that genetic factors are involved in obesity.

However, social factors interact with genetic factors in determining body fatness. This is indicated by the observation that in affluent societies both children and adults from the lower income classes are more likely to be overweight (Black 1983), and the prevalence of overweight was higher amongst girls, but not boys, from lower socio-economic groups (Peckham *et al.* 1983).

ENERGY INTAKE

Individual energy requirement varies widely from the mean recommended allowances for any age or weight, and depends in part on energy expenditure and growth.

Recent surveys by Whitehead *et al.* (1981) and McKillop & Durnin (1982) have shown that many infants who were growing normally had lower energy intakes than recommended allowances suggest. The individual differences in energy intake of children is evident from birth and no relationship can be found between amounts of milk taken, size, adiposity or rate of weight gain (Morgan & Mumford 1981).

Parental eating habits are superimposed on the child, both regarding type and quantity of food. However, the traditional view that overweight subjects eat more or exercise less is not uniformly true. Children with higher energy intakes are not necessarily the most active. Normal weight children aged 4 to 5 years with one obese parent consumed 20% less energy than an equivalent group of children who had normal weight parents (Griffiths & Payne

1976). Such findings suggest that low energy requirements predispose to obesity and familial obesity may have a metabolic as well as a social basis (Black 1983). Griffiths & Payne (1976) found the children from obese families had a lower metabolic rate and a lower estimated energy expenditure than the children from normal weight families. As yet no hormonal basis for the metabolic susceptibility to weight gain has been found. Hampton et al. (1967) studied the energy intake in 11- to 15-year-olds and found those who were overweight had lower energy intakes for both lean body weight and total body weight compared to the non-obese.

Adjustment of energy intake for energy expenditure is neither immediate nor precise. Control of food intake in man is complex. Fomon et al. (1969, 1971) studied the intake of infants offered different energy density feeds. The mothers were unaware that the energy density of the milk was being altered and were encouraged to allow the child to decide on his or her own intake. The babies offered feeds with half the normal energy density quickly increased their intake but only to approximately 80% rather than the 100% needed for precise compensation. This inability to compensate completely seemed particularly marked in the first month of life, 1 of the 9 children failing to compensate to any appreciable extent. However, the older infants in some way acquired the ability to recognize and compensate for the dilutions in the energy density of the milks. Older malnourished children in Jamaica (Ashworth 1974) following an infection, after the first few days of treatment, developed a voracious appetite and if allowed to ingest an energy dense milk took twice as much energy intake on a weight basis than usual and grew at 15 times the normal rate until they attained an appropriate weight for height. At this point the amount of food ingested usually fell abruptly, within 48 hours, to an intake normally expected in a child of that size. This pattern was also observed in children on mixed diets.

Studies summarized by Black (1983) with different energy density diets in adults on the regulation of energy intake have confirmed that any physiological adjustment in energy intake takes several days to occur, there being no instant response to the change in body energy stores. Regulating systems can sense as little as 25% energy reduction and the compensatory response limited the energy deficit to less than 15% of the habitual energy intake (Black 1983). If precise control operates body weight will not vary, however the slow changes in body weight seen in adults suggests energy regulation systems controlling intake and expenditure are not very accurate but do exist. The physiological mechanisms by which man adjusts his intake also involve psychological factors such as taste, colour and texture allowing a link between sensory attributes and energy content to be established. A larger variety of different foods encourages a higher energy intake than a limited range of food.

Recent evidence in animal studies suggests that there are specific appetite drives with the animal selecting foods in order to obtain an appropriate intake of vitamins, minerals, protein and carbohydrate, and that powerful controls operate to maintain an intake of nutrients in the most suitable proportions (cited in Black 1983). No evidence in man is available, but it is unwise to assume that those who demonstrate unusual patterns of food intake do so solely as a result of emotional factors.

When presented with increasing concentrations of glucose, food preferences can be observed from birth. Thin babies show an aversion to sweet solutions in contrast to fat babies. These differences may in part reflect the physiological effects of body composition at birth but they may also be innate (Rodin 1981).

The interaction between mother and child is also very important and the learning of food habits can mean that some children are trained to eat more than their physiological needs.

Artificial feeding of infants and the early introduction of solids can lead more easily to excess energy intake causing rapid weight gain in infancy, compared to breast-feeding (Taitz 1971). Rose & Mayer (1968) found thin infants tend to eat less and be more active. The trend to obesity may start at an early age (Brook et al. 1972), particularly where there is a genetic predisposition to obesity (Court & Dunlop 1975).

A diet composed largely of high energy density foods such as those rich in fat and sugar makes it relatively easy to consume a high energy intake particularly when such foods are made desirable by family food habits, peer group pressures and extensive advertising by the media. Those individuals who are metabolically most susceptible to weight gain will be at greatest risk.

Excess energy intake compared to expenditure need not be great to cause excess weight gain; 420 kJ (100 kcal) per day in excess of requirement, theoretically causes a 4.5 kg (10 lb) weight gain per year); likewise, the reverse can be true, although various other factors come into play. An energy value of 420 kJ (100 kcal) is contained in one slice of bread and butter, 2 small boiled potatoes, 20 g ($\frac{2}{3}$ oz) chocolate or crisps, or one ice-cream brickette.

PHYSICAL ACTIVITY

Physical inactivity may contribute to the development of obesity in the community and a decline in activity levels will mean that those who are susceptible to weight gain will be at risk. However, what determines the spontaneous physical activity in children is uncertain (Black 1983). In general, physical activity involves an increase in energy expenditure and is therefore likely to limit weight gain, however subsequent alteration in food intake and physical activity at other times may counteract the effect of vigorous exercise. Studies in children in the UK suggest there has been a decrease in both energy intake and expenditure over recent years. The reduced dietary energy intake has not always been sufficient compensation to prevent fat accumulation. Whether patients who are overweight utilize energy differently, or whether their reduced physical activity alone accounts for reduced dietary needs is not clear. Individuals who are obese tend to move less quickly than the lean and expend less energy in sitting, standing and walking even before they become obese (Craddock 1982), i.e., reduced activity was thought to be a cause of, rather than result of, overweight. The daily energy expenditure at rest was appreciably less, and energy expenditure with activity was shown to be reduced in children who were overweight when starting school in the study by Griffiths & Payne (1976), and in teenagers by Anderson (1972). However many studies fail to take into account the greater physical cost of exercise in the obese (Garrow 1974).

Physical activity has probably decreased with social change in the affluent society. Children may get less exercise due to high-rise flats isolating them from play grounds and giving only small areas for play, buses and cars now frequently take children to school if it is any distance from home, and increased environmental temperature and clothing decrease energy requirements.

Gwinup (1975) demonstrated that exercise alone could achieve weight loss in a small group of women who were obese taking regular exercise for 30+ minutes a day but those with the greatest weight loss were taking ≥ 3 hours exercise daily. Exercise alone as a means of weight loss is not advocated but increased activity on a regular basis should be encouraged, especially in children in conjunction with a change in diet.

Team games are usually unpopular with children who are overweight as they become embarrassed about their appearance and clumsiness. Running, skipping and swimming are particularly useful; even walking which uses approximately 1300 kJ (300 kcal) per hour should be encouraged.

PSYCHOLOGICAL AND SOCIAL FACTORS

Social, psychological, endocrinological, and metabolic factors all contribute to the prevalence of overweight in the community as a whole, and several factors may be involved in any individual who is overweight. Secular changes in Britain have affected eating habits, social patterns and physical activity which may favour weight gain in the population (Black 1983). Energy intake can easily exceed expenditure when food availability permits people to eat all they desire and few take enough exercise.

Overweight carries a social stigma and often children are made a figure of fun and are thought responsible for their condition. A feeling of personal shame frequently occurs as a result of such condemnation and rejection particularly in the adolescent who is overweight. Those involved in management should not imply overweight patients are self-indulgent or lack will-power (Black 1983).

Various psychocultural factors can lead to overeating. The majority find eating a pleasure; contentment and eating are closely related to mother-child relationships. Children quickly learn to eat in order to please their mother, whilst others use meal times and food as a weapon. Parents frequently reward children materially, food rewards are common and are used for comfort with the result that food is used as a comfort in times of stress.

Overweight is less common in both sexes in the upper compared to the lower social classes and those who move up the social scale tend to lose thier overweight. This is apparent even in children (Whitelaw 1971; Peckham *et al.* 1983).

Primary emotional factors in the parent or child can result in over-compensation with food, e.g., by parents of the emotionally deprived, mentally retarded or physically handicapped child. Overeating may be precipitated by an emotional crisis such as the death of a parent, separation of parents, or failure in examinations (Anderson 1972), which can result in overweight. Overweight is more common in only children (Whitelaw 1971) and in children from one parent homes (Wilkinson *et al.* 1977). Dieting and isolation from peer group either because of overweight or its treatment can cause secondary psychological problems.

PHYSIOLOGY

Controversy still continues over whether the number of adipose tissue cells can be increased by overfeeding (Craddock 1982; Black 1983). It is most probable that their number is genetically determined (Chlouverakis 1974). The number increases rapidly in infants and more slowly thereafter until the mid-teens. In adults the increased volume of adipose tissue is brought about by increased size in existing cells rather than an increase in number, and a loss of weight results in a decrease in their size (Häger 1977).

METABOLIC AND ENDOCRINOLOGICAL FACTORS

The difference in body fat content between males and females is small until adolescence. Women have a body fat content of 20 to 25% whereas in men it is only 12 to 17% of their weight. However the average basal metabolic rate per unit of total body weight is similar in both men and women (Black 1983).

Metabolic abnormalities most commonly occur in severe obesity; they tend to become abnormal with time but are reversible with weight loss. Insulin levels are increased and correlate with the degree of obesity (Lestradet *et al.* 1975), but are decreased with exercise even when weight loss is not achieved (Björntorp 1978). Elevated fasting blood sugar levels are found and correlate with an increase in blood pressure (Florey *et al.* 1976).

Height velocity is accelerated from the onset of excess weight gain. However growth tends to stop at an earlier age, such that the final height of the adult who was overweight as a child is only slightly higher than average (Forbes 1977).

The vast majority of patients who are overweight have no clinical evidence of an endocrine disorder. Overweight, however, frequently accompanies certain rare endocrine disorders such as Cushing's syndrome, hypothyroidism and some pituitary abnormalities. The most frequent of these conditions is Prader-Willi syndrome which occurs in approximately 1 in 20 000 births. These congenital disorders are characterized by short stature in contrast to those who have 'simple' overweight. The metabolic basis of overweight in these conditions remains uncertain. The overweight accompanying these conditions responds to restriction in energy intake.

Prader-Willi syndrome is of particular interest as it has been considered an intractable form of obesity with onset from 1 to 4 years of age and is a lifelong problem. Patients have a craving for food. Paradoxically feeding difficulties and even poor growth are features of the infant. Weight reduction is said to require severe restriction of energy intake and has been consistently unsuccessful. However rigorous control of energy intake can achieve appropriate control of weight to permit maximal potential of these patients. A prevention regimen has been reported by Pipes & Holm (1973) which with parental support has been found successful. A parents support group has been formed recently.

TREATMENT AND MANAGEMENT OF OVERWEIGHT

The increased risk of overweight children becoming overweight or obese adults necessitates intervention. Even though the majority will achieve more appropriate proportions, a substantial number will remain overweight or become overweight again in adult life. If overweight persists into adult life fat accumulation can become extreme (Black 1983).

The risk of anorexia nervosa developing in adolescent girls who attempt to slim should not be dismissed, but is probably over exaggerated and should not deter from sensible advice being given about eating and weight gain, which need modification on a long-term basis in those who are overweight.

A detailed history of food and environmental factors surrounding food intake and the family is essential. Pregnancy record, family history, weight gain in infancy, onset of excess weight gain and the child's eating habits are all relevant. To be successful, the child from school age onwards must want to lose weight, but requires support and co-operation from the parents or guardian and ideally the whole family unit. It is important to establish whether the food intake and exercise pattern are unusual or relatively low, particularly as children of overweight parents have an increased risk of overweight and tend to have lower energy needs than average.

Assessment of weight gain in children depends in part on growth and therefore the child's height, weight and skinfold measurements in at least the triceps and abdominal area should be taken and used to monitor success of any intervention programme. These should be recorded on percentile charts.

INFANTS

The diet of overweight infants under 6 months of age should not normally be restricted and older infants and toddlers should merely have their diet modified to slow down weight gain. However these 'at risk' infants should be supervised and their parents given appropriate advice in order to develop sensible eating habits based on normal nutrition, so that subsequent overweight is prevented. The following have been found helpful in correcting excess weight gain in infants:

1.   Support of the mother in handling the child and guiding her in interpreting his or her needs, e.g., some limitation of suckling time in the breast-fed infant may be needed.

2.   Correct feed dilution in an appropriate volume for age should be advised. Once a range of solids are introduced at 3 meal times, milk intake should be limited to approximately 500 ml (1 pint) per day.

3.   Avoidance of added sugar to feeds and solids.

4.   Avoidance of cereals and solids added to bottle feeds.

5.   Water should be offered for drinking rather than sweetened drinks and the use of 'dinky' feeders discouraged. Some natural fruit juice, diluted and unsweetened, can be offered once-daily from about 3 months old.

6.   The use of a dummy or water to drink after feeds to comfort the child and provide adequate sucking can be helpful.

7.   A small-holed teat should be used for bottle feeds to slow down drinking time and weaning off the bottle at about 8 months and before 1 year of age is advisable as infants usually take less volume of feed from a cup or 'teacher beaker' than bottle.

8.   Added fat and high energy density solids should be avoided and substituted with lower energy density high nutrient foods such as fruit, vegetables, wholegrain cereals, low fat fish and lean meats.

9.   Supplements of vitamin A, D, C are advised.

CHILDREN

The actual treatment of overweight depends on the age of the child and degree of overweight. Over-restricted diets that inhibit growth should be avoided but some dietary control from onset or pre-school age is essential to long-term success. It may be desirable either to reduce the weight or allow the child to 'grow into his or her actual weight' by maintaining a steady weight until this is appropriate for age, height and sex and the child has achieved more appropriate proportions. In the pre-school age child the latter is usually advised. In theory this is simple, but in practice difficult and long-term results even in children are often discouraging (Stark et al. 1975). Prevention of overweight from early childhood is therefore of prime importance. The younger the child, the more likely is the chance of changing the dietary pattern, changing the dietary energy density and so reducing overweight, or changing the state of energy balance to a more satisfactory level. Success is most likely if the whole family is involved in the new pattern of eating, and the parents (and child once old enough) are motivated and have a genuine desire for the child to lose weight, understand the hazards of overweight, how it has occurred, and are re-educated about a well-balanced and varied diet of reduced energy intake. Selective dieting of overweight children within the family may lead to a feeling of isolation and deprivation, particularly if a very restricted diet is suggested which is inadvisable for a number of reasons.

Ditschuneit et al. (1978) showed that on a 'free' diet excluding snacks, sugar, white flour and reduced fat intake, but allowing ample quantities of natural basic foods containing protein, minerals and vitamins (see food groups Table 1.11) energy intake was reduced and weight loss could be achieved. Such a diet allows unlimited lean meat, fish, fruit, vegetables, wholegrain cereals and wholemeal bread, e.g., 200 g (7 oz) per day with an intake of skimmed milk, e.g., 500 ml (1 pint) per day, and butter or margarine, e.g., 30 g (1 oz) per day. Low energy sugar-free drinks and artificial sweeteners are permitted.

Dietary Treatment for Overweight Children

In moderate to severe overweight, the previous dietary intake should be assessed and a suitable reduced energy intake advised. The diet advised varies but is frequently in the range of 3500 kJ to 6000 kJ (800 to 1450 kcal) per day in school age children and 8500 kJ (2000 kcal) during adolescence. Examples are given in Table 2.1. In children not less than a daily intake of 26 kJ (6 kcal) per cm height in females and 35 kJ (8 kcal) per cm height in males should be recommended, which is approximately 50% of the energy requirement for normal children (Beal 1970). Adequate variety,

Table 2.1 Quantity of food for various restricted energy diets for children.

	3500 kJ (800 kcal)	4000 kJ (1000 kcal)	5000 kJ (1200 kcal)	6000 kJ (1450 kcal)
1 Lean meat, egg, cheese, fish Poultry, bacon, offal Grilled sausage, beefburger, fish fingers Luncheon meat, corned beef May be steamed, grilled, roast, braised, boiled. Lean only, not fried	2 × 50 g serving = 1000 kJ (240 kcal)	3 × 50 g serving = 1500 kJ (360 kcal)	3 × 50 g serving = 1500 kJ (360 kcal)	3 × 50 g serving = 1500 kJ (360 kcal)
2 Bread, medium slices (40g) preferably wholemeal or exchanges of potato and cereal (see **Table 2.2**)	1½ slices = 600 kJ (150 kcal)	1½ slices = 600 kJ (150 kcal)	3½ slices = 1400 kJ (350 kcal)	5 slices = 2000 kJ (500 kcal)
3 Butter or margarine[a] or double quantity of low fat spread[a], e.g. Outline	15 g = 200 kJ (50 kcal)	15 g = 200 kJ (50 kcal)	15 g = 200 kJ (50 kcal)	30 g = 400 g kJ (100 kcal)

4 Skimmed milk, or exchanges (See **Table 2.3**)	800 ml = 1100 kJ (260 kcal)	800 ml = 1100 kJ (260 kcal)	800 ml = 1000 kJ (260 kcal)	800 ml = 1100 kJ (260 kcal)
5 Fruit, average size apple, orange, pear, peach or 2 mandarins or 80 g grapes or ½ banana or average serving unsweetened stewed fruit or 1 serving unsweetened tinned fruit or 1 glass natural fruit juice unsweetened, or 1 large grapefruit.	2 servings = 400 kJ (100 kcal)	3 servings = 600 kJ (150 kcal)	3 servings = 600 kJ (150 kcal)	4 servings = 800 kJ (200 kcal)
6 Root vegetables, peas, beetroot	1 serving = 100 kJ (25 kcal)	1 serving = 100 kJ (25 kcal)	1 serving = 100 kJ (25 kcal)	1 serving = 100 kJ (25 kcal)
Total	3400 kJ (825 kcal)	4100 kJ (995 kcal)	4900 kJ (1195 kcal)	5900 kJ (1445 kcal)

[a] High in Poly Unsaturated Fatty Acids

Low energy foods (see pp. 108–10) are permitted freely in addition

Children's Vitamin A, D, C, Drops (Welfare Food Supplies) or 0.6 ml Abidec (Parke Davis).

protein, fibre, vitamins, minerals and bulk should be included in the regimen.

There is even less evidence in children than adults that very low energy diets are beneficial and they may prove harmful since not only does linear growth cease but the smaller reserves of lean tissue in a child places him or her at increased risk of tissue depletion and illness (Black 1983). On such diets metabolic rate is decreased, the diet does not prepare for long-term diet modification, and often the diet is 'sensibly disregarded'. Such diets are low in utilizable protein for growth, fibre, mineral and vitamin content and lack variety. Starvation and protein supplemented fasts are never appropriate in children and diets of less than 3500 kJ (800 kcal) are rarely advisable.

In children who have become accustomed to food for comfort, the inclusion of a restricted intake of a 'treat' food as a reward either daily, weekly or both as appropriate can be important psychologically, and can be used to help motivate the child to continue the diet. The energy intake provided from such items should be taken into account in the total dietary regimen.

The dietary aim should allow the child enough food to avoid real hunger, which only encourages pilfering, and yet achieve a small steady weight loss. Theoretically 1 kg (2 lb) weight loss requires a deficit of 4200 kJ (1000 kcal), as the energy value of obese tissue is about 31 kJ (7.5 kcal) per g. Such a deficit of energy is considerable for school age and younger children, and therefore 1 to 2 kg (2 to 4 lb) weight loss per month is the recommended aim and diets should be planned accordingly. Weight should be checked initially at not more frequently than weekly intervals, and once weight loss has started at 4-weekly intervals. Height should be measured at approximately 3-monthly intervals together with skinfold measurements. It is helpful if these are recorded on growth percentile charts to which the patient has access.

Some patients appear to lack the sensation of satiety; the child with Prader-Willi syndrome is the extreme example (Pipes & Holm 1973). The aim is to suppress hunger by the inclusion of large quantities of high bulk, lower energy density foods such as wholegrain cereals, fruit and vegetables which are rich in fibre. Low energy (calorie) soups or drinks taken with meals can be used to provide variety and 'extend' meals. Previous suggestions that protein foods provide satiety have been questioned. Fibre supplements alone are ineffective (McLean & Baird 1978), though an increase of wholegrain cereals and the use of wholemeal bread are recommended and help prevent constipation which in the past often accompanied dieting. Concentrated energy foods containing refined sugar and large quantities of fats should usually be avoided. Overweight children frequently dislike vegetables, fruit, wholegrain cereals and even plain meat dishes, having grown accustomed to snack foods and convenience foods which are high in energy, carbohydrate and fat. Correction of these food habits takes a great deal of persuasion and perseverance; compromise is frequently necessary, at least initially.

Social support of the family by the general practitioner, health visitor, paediatrician and/or dietitian as an adjunct to diet modification is essential. Group therapy and psychological support may be helpful in achieving weight loss in overweight children as well as adults.

Behaviour modification methods to achieve weight loss in adults have proved disappointing as a means of changing eating habits in the long-term and maintenance of weight loss beyond one year is less than satisfactory. All long-term studies have found that weight increases again in the majority treated for obesity with behaviour modification alone (Stunkard & Penick 1979). Further evaluation is needed before it can be recommended for general use or in children.

As an adjunct to dietary advice it may be helpful to encourage eating more slowly in those who eat quickly, e.g., by replacing cutlery or finger foods onto the plate between mouthfuls. Care is needed so as not to reinforce inappropriate behaviour, e.g., attention seeking. If praise and reward schemes are used to motivate the child, suitable rewards must be devised, parental support given and careful follow-up is necessary to check that desirable results are achieved. Physical activity and exercise should be encouraged in all children and particularly as an adjunct to dietary modification in children who are overweight.

QUALITATIVE MODIFICATION OF DIET

An acceptable palatable and nutritionally adequate diet is essential. Qualitative modifications of diet, apart from obvious sugar and fat restrictions, make little or no difference to weight loss compared to a simple reduction in total energy. Low carbohydrate diets which severely limit starch and unrefined carbohydrates are inappropriate on general nutritional principles. Rapid weight loss occurs, with a diuresis and loss of muscle glycogen followed by the development of ketosis. Although the ketosis may suppress the ketosis may suppress appetite, such diets may not correct the accompanying hyperlipidaemia which occurs with obesity. High fat diets for weight loss should be strongly discouraged if the risk of coronary heart disease which is associated with overweight in adults is not to be exacerbated (Black 1983). Protein supplemented fasts are not appropriate. High protein regimens are not recommended as they are also high in fat and are expensive.

Slimming foods for meal replacement usually have a basic energy content of 4200 kJ (1000 kcal) per day, but little is known of their long-term effect, particularly in children. They lack variety and do nothing towards educating the patient to a more appropriate balanced meal pattern.

Slimming biscuits contain more energy than ordinary plain biscuits, and many 'diabetic' products have a higher energy value than the conventional product as the usual sugar is simply replaced by sorbitol or fructose and may have a higher fat content such as in 'diabetic' chocolate. Sorbitol ($C_6H_{14}O_6$) is a sugar-like substance which breaks down in the body to produce energy. The energy value of sorbitol and fructose are similar to sugar and glucose in the diet which renders them inappropriate in diets aimed to reduce weight. Sorbitol is the basis of many powdered sweeteners and others contain lactose, fructose, manose and other sugars, therefore this type of powdered sweetener should be discouraged in energy restricted diets, though the high sweetness value of some products reduces the total quantity taken and so marginally helps reduce energy intake.

Saccharine and its derivatives in liquid or tablet form can be used in moderation for sweetening foods as these are inert chemicals which do not release energy in the body, and due to their high sweetness value are used in very small quantities. Several new chemical sweeteners which are more palatable then saccharine and energy free have become available recently such as aspartame and acesulfame-potassium. They are now being used extensively to sweeten low-calorie drinks and desserts. Excess use of any sweetener should, however, be discouraged as it is preferable that the child loses the appeal for sweet-tasting food.

APPETITE SUPPRESSANT DRUGS: DIETHYLPROPION, FENFLURAMINE, MAZINDOL AND PHENTERMINE

The majority of obese patients report appetite suppressant drugs are useful in helping them to adhere to a low energy diet in order to lose weight, particularly in the initial stage of slimming. Anorectic drugs are effective but growth velocity may be impaired in children (Rayner & Court 1975). Some physicians use a drug such as diethylpropion as a support to energy controlled diets in children who find it difficult to lose weight (Craddock 1982). It must be monitored and stopped if growth or weight loss stops and physicians should be aware that psychological dependence on the drug can occasionally occur. These drugs should only be used as an additional therapy to dietary modification.

SOCIAL EATING

Social aspects of a diet should not be overlooked. School lunch may be supplied either as a home-prepared packed lunch of sandwiches and fruit, or the savoury course of the traditional school dinner is permitted with replacement of pudding or dessert with fresh fruit. Children of families who are entitled to free school dinners should be encouraged to take advantage of this service. Liaison with school meal organizers and appropriate adjustment of the remaining dietary intake is usually a satisfactory means of devising an appropriate regimen.

Tea with friends, with a little forethought and liaison with the parent or guardian regarding suitable menus, can be a pleasurable experience for the child. A picnic including a low energy (calorie-free) drink and a special treat can be the highlight to a family outing.

FOLLOW-UP

Dietary modification should continue until the child's weight is satisfactory and in proportion for both height and age. Care should then be taken to slowly introduce a more liberal diet based on normal nutrition and the child taught how to maintain an appropriate weight, otherwise return to the old meal pattern frequently results in weight being regained. Follow-up and support is essential; even so, long-term results are disappointing (Lloyd *et al.* 1977). The family, or child if old enough, should be encouraged to have the child's height and weight measured regularly at approximately 3-monthly intervals, recorded on growth percentile charts so that the family can take appropriate action or precautions as soon as weight gain becomes inappropriate.

LOW ENERGY DIET FOR TREATMENT OF OVERWEIGHT IN CHILDREN

Basic foods selected from the food groups (Table 1.11) such as meat, fruit, vegetables, milk and bread (preferably wholemeal) are included to provide a high nutrient density of protein, vitamins, fibre and minerals in the low energy diet. The quantity of these foods can be unlimited as in the 'free' diet or restricted to the energy intake required, as individually calculated or as suggested in the examples in Table 2.1. Bread exchanges of similar energy value are given in Table 2.2, and milk exchanges in Table 2.3. Vitamin supplements, as Children's Vitamin A, D, C, Drops or Abidec 0.6 ml for under 5-year-olds or a more comprehensive supplement of vitamins and minerals can be prescribed as appropriate. A sample menu is given in Table 2.4 as a guide for a low energy dietary regimen.

LOW ENERGY FOODS ALLOWED FREELY

Low energy foods are allowed freely in addition to the foods listed in Table 2.1 and should be encouraged to provide bulk, trace

Table 2.2   Bread exchanges based on energy value (approx. 400 kJ/100 kcal).

Bread and Biscuits	40 g	Bread, 1 medium slice, use wholemeal for preference
	25 g	Crispbread
	20 g	Cream crackers/water biscuits
	20 g	Semi-sweet or digestive biscuits
	50 g	Chapati cooked without fat
	25 g	Chapati cooked with fat
Cereals, unsweetened		Use wholegrain types for preference
	30 g	Allbran
	25 g	Weetabix (1 biscuit)
	25 g	Museli
	25 g	Shredded Wheat
	25 g	Cornflakes
	25 g	Rice Krispies
Potatoes	100 g	Boiled or jacket potato (2 small)
	100 g	Mashed potato, 2 small scoops
	60 g	Roast potato, 1 medium
	30 g	Chips, 6 medium
	15 g	Crisps, 1 small packet
Miscellaneous	150 g	Baked beans (1 small tin)
	150 g	Spaghetti, in tomato sauce (1 small tin)
	75 g	Boiled rice

nutrients and variety in the diet. These include:

Vegetables

All greens: french and runner beans, cabbage, cauliflower, broccoli, spinach, sprouts, spring greens, courgettes, aubergine

Salads: lettuce, tomato, cucumber, cress, celery, radish, spring onion, chinese cabbage

Onions, leeks, mushrooms (not fried), marrow, asparagus, peppers, swede, turnip, carrot, parsnip, peas and beetroot *in moderation*

Parsley, mint, chives

Beverages

Water

Tea or coffee made with milk from daily allowance (may be sweetened with saccharine or aspartame etc.).

Low energy (calorie) or dietetic fruit squash/drink

Natural unsweetened fruit juice in moderation, e.g., 1 glass daily

Sugarless carbonated drinks, e.g., Trim Slimline, OneCal, Diet Pepsi, Tab etc.

Unsweetened lemon juice, tomato or grapefruit juice, soda water

Clear soups and broth, stock cubes

Unthickened gravy with fat removed

Marmite, Oxo, Bovril. Bisto-type gravy

Miscellaneous

Salt, pepper, herbs, spices, curry powder, vinegar, clear pickles

Bran

Worcester sauce, brown sauce, ketchup and tomato sauce *in moderation*

Flavouring, essences, e.g., vanilla

Sweeteners such as saccharine, aspartame, acesulfame-potassium in tablet or liquid form

Rennet, powderd gelatine and sugarless jellies

Table 2.3 100 ml Milk exchanges based on energy value (approx. 270 kJ/60 kcal).

100 ml	Milk, whole or full fat
150 ml	Reduced (2%) fat milk (semi-skimmed)
200 ml	Skimmed milk
20 g	Skimmed milk powder
60 g	Cottage cheese
15 g	Cheddar cheese
120 g	Natural low fat yoghurt
75 g	Fruit or flavoured low fat yoghurt
40 g	Ice-cream, plain varieties

Table 2.4 Low energy (calorie) diet example menu[a].

Daily	. . . milk allowance Children's Vitamin A, C, D, Drops or 0.6 ml Abidec
Breakfast	Fruit, e.g., ½ grapefruit . . . unsweetened cereal Milk from allowance Egg, boiled or poached **or** bacon, grilled **or** ham and tomatoes **or** fish Tea or coffee (no sugar) . . . bread (may be toasted), preferably wholemeal Scraping of butter or margarine[b], or low fat spread[b]
Mid-morning	Milk from allowance or low energy/calorie fruit squash/drink
Lunch/Dinner	Average serving lean meat and gravy **or** fish **Or** small serving first . . . potato course school dinner 1 serving peas or root vegetable and 1 piece fruit in Greens or other vegetable from free list place of pudding/ . . . fruit dessert
Tea	Low calorie fruit squash/drink or tea with milk (no sugar) Bread exchange if permitted with scraping butter or margarine[b], or low fat spread[b]
Supper/ High Tea	1 serving lean meat, fish, cheese or egg Salad or green vegetables . . . bread (and scraping butter) or bread exchange . . . fruit Remaining milk from allowance or cup of tea or milk exchange

[a] The appropriate quantities for milk, bread, fruit and potato are calculated according to the energy value of the diet required.
[b] High in Poly Unsaturated Fatty Acids.

Low energy (calorie) salad dressing; other 'slimming' salad creams in moderation
Sugarless pastilles and sugarless chewing gum

HIGH ENERGY FOOD LIMITATIONS

High energy foods which should be avoided or used in strict limitation for treats. These foods are **not** necessary for health.

Concentrated carbohydrates
Sugar, glucose, jam, honey, marmalade, syrup, treacle, sweets, chocolate, lollies, ice lollies
Sweetened squash, fruit juices, fizzy drinks

Cakes, biscuits, pastries, sweetened cereals
Puddings
Fruit
Sweetened tinned fruit, jelly
Dried fruit and nuts except *in moderation*
Soups and sauces
Sweet pickles and chutneys, thick soup, tinned and packet soups
Thick sauces and gravies
Beverages
Sweetened chocolate drinks, milk shake syrups and powders, drinking chocolate, malted milks
Alcoholic beverages
Concentrated fats
Cooking fats and oil
Salad dressing, salad cream, mayonnaise
All fried foods
Liver paté, fatty sausages, black pudding, salami, goose, duck
Visible fat on meat
Cream
Miscellaneous
Sorbitol, powdered artificial sweeteners
'Diabetic' products such as chocolate, jam, biscuits
'Slimming' biscuits and similar products

USEFUL ADDRESS

Prader-Willi Syndrome Parents Association
30 Follett Drive
Abbots Langley
Herts WD5 0LP

REFERENCES

ABRAHAM A., COLLINS G. & NORDSIECK M. (1971) Relationship of childhood weight status to morbidity in adults. *HSMHA Health Reports* **86**, 73.
ANDERSON J. (1972) Obesity. *British Medical Journal* **1**, 560.
ASHWORTH A. (1974) Ad-lib feeding during recovery from malnutrition. *British Medical Journal of Nutrition* **31**, 109.
BEAL V. A. (1970) Nutritional intake. In McCammon R. W. (ed.). *Human Growth and Development*, p.61. Charles C. Thomas, Springfield, Illinois.

112 Chapter 2

BJÖRNTORP P. (1978) Physical training in the treatment of obesity. *International Journal of Obesity* **2**, 249.

BLACK, SIR DOUGLAS (Chairman) (1983) Obesity. *Journal of the Royal College of Physicians of London* **17**, 5–65.

BRAY G. A. (1981) The inheritance of corpulence. In Cioffi L. A., James W. P. T. & Van Itallie T. B. (eds) *The Bodyweight Regulatory System: Normal and Disturbed Mechanisms*, pp.185–95. Raven, New York.

BROOK C. G. D. (1971) Determinations of body composition of children from skinfold measurements. *Archives of Disease in Childhood* **46**, 182.

BROOK C. G. D. (1974) In Burland W. L., Samuel P. D. & Yudkin J. (eds) *Obesity*, p.86. Churchill Livingstone, Edinburgh.

BROOK C. G. D., LLOYD J. K. & WOLFF O. H. (1972) Relation between age of onset of obesity and size and number of adipose cells. *British Medical Journal* **2**, 25.

CHLOUVERAKIS C. S. (1974) Controversies in medicine (iv)—regulation of adipose tissue mass. *Obesity/Bariatric Medicine* **3**, 86.

COURT J. M. & DUNLOP M. (1975) In Howard A. (ed) *Recent Advances in Obesity Research*, p.34. Newman, London.

CRADDOCK D. (1978) *Obesity and its Management*, 3rd ed., p.13. Churchill Livingstone, Edinburgh.

CRADDOCK D. (1982) Obesity. In McLaren D. S. & Burman D. (eds) *Textbook of Paediatric Nutrition*, 2nd ed., pp.191–205. Churchill Livingstone, Edinburgh.

DHSS/MRC (1976) *Report on Research on Obesity* (compiled by James W. P. T.). HMSO, London.

DHSS (1983, revised) *Present Day Practice in Infant Feeding*, Report No. 20, 1980. HMSO, London.

DITSCHUNEIT H. H., JUNG F. & DITSCHUNEIT H. (1978) Treatment of obese children with a low carbohydrate protein rich diet. *International Journal of Obesity* **2**, 476.

FLOREY C., DU V., UPPAL S. & LOWEY C. (1976) Relation between blood pressure, weight and plasma sugar and serum insulin levels in school children aged 9 to 12 years in Westland, Holland. *British Medical Journal* **1**, 1368.

FOMON S. J., FILER L. J., THOMAS L. N., ROGER R. R. & PROKSCH A. M. (1969) Relationship between formula concentration and rate of growth of normal children. *Journal of Nutrition* **198**, 241.

FOMON S. J., THOMAS L. N., FILER L. J., ZIEGLER E. E. & LEONARD M. T. (1971) Food consumption and growth of normal infants fed milk-based formulae. *Acta Paediatrica Scandinavica* Supplement **223**, 1–36.

FORBES G. B. (1977) Nutrition and Growth. *Journal of Pediatrics* **91**, 40.

FRANCIS D. E. M. (1974) Low calorie diets for obesity. In Francis D. E. M. *Diets for Sick Children*, 3rd edn. Blackwell Scientific Publications, Oxford.

GARN S. M. & CLARK D. C. (1976) Trends in fatness and the origins of obesity. *Pediatrics* **57**, 443.

Garrow J. S. (1974) *Energy Balance and Obesity in Man.* North Holland Publishing Company, Amsterdam.

Garrow J. S. (1978) *Energy Balance and Obesity in Man,* 2nd ed. Elsevier, Amsterdam.

Griffiths M. & Payne P. R. (1976) Energy expenditure in small children of obese and non-obese parents. *Nature* **260,** 698.

Gwinup G. (1975) Effects of exercise alone on the weight of obese women. *Archives of International Medicine* **135,** 676–80.

Häger, A. (1977) Adipose cell size and number in relation to obesity. *Postgraduate Medical Journal* **53,** (suppl. 2), 101.

Hampton M. C., Huenemann R. L., Shapiro L. R., et al. (1966) A longitudinal study of gross body composition and body conformation and their association with food and activity in a teenage population. Anthropometric evaluation of body fluid. *American Journal of Clinical Nutrition* **19,** 422–35.

Lestradet H., Deschamps I., Giron B. & Ostrowski Z. L. (1975) Relationship between the size of adipocytes, blood glucose, plasma insulin, non esterfied fatty acids and the degree of obesity in children. In Howard A. (ed.) *Recent Advances in Obesity Research,* p.167. Newman, London.

Lloyd J. K. (1977) Prognosis of obesity in infancy and childhood. *Postgraduate Medical Journal* **53,** (suppl. 2), 111.

McLean D. S. & Baird I. (1978) Obesity and anorexia nervosa. In Dickerson J. W. T. & Lee J. A. (eds) *Nutrition in Clinical Management of Disease,* pp.105–17. Edward Arnold, London.

McKillop F. M. & Durnin J. V. G.A. (1982) The energy and nutrition intake of a random sample (305) of infants. *Human Nutrition: Applied Nutrition* **36A,** 405–21.

Morgan J. & Mumford P. (1981) Preliminary studies of energy expenditure in infants under 6 months of age. *Acta Paediatrica Scandinavica* **70,** 15.

Peckham C. S., Stark O., Simonite V. & Wolff O. H. (1983) Prevalence of obesity in British children born in 1946 and 1958. *British Medical Journal* **286,** 1237–42.

Pipes P. L. & Holm V. A. (1973) Weight control of children with Prader-Willi Syndrome. *Journal of the American Dietetic Association* **62,** 520–4.

Poskitt E. M. E. & Cole T. J. (1977) Do fat babies stay fat? *British Medical Journal* **1,** 7–9.

Rayner P. & Court J. (1975) Effects of dietary restriction and anorectic drugs on linear growth in childhood obesity. *Archives of Disease in Childhood* **49,** 821.

Rodin J. (1981) Psychological factors in obesity. In Björntorp P., Carilla M. & Howard A. N. (eds) *Recent Advances in Obesity Research III.* John Libbey, London.

Rose H. E. & Mayer J. (1968) Activity, calorie intake, fat storage and energy balance of infants. *Pediatrics* **41,** 15.

SHUKLA A., FORSYTHE H. A., ANDERSON C. M. & MARWAH S. M. (1972) Infantile overnutrition in the first year of life. *British Medical Journal* **4,** 507–15.

STARK O., LLOYD J. K. & WOLFF O. H. (1975) Long term results of hospital in-patient treatment of obese children. In Howard A. (ed.) *Recent Advances in Obesity Research,* p.289. Newman, London.

STARK O., ATKINS E., WOLFF O. H. & DOUGLAS J. W. B. (1981) Longitudinal study of obesity in the National Survey of Health and Development. *British Medical Journal* **283,** 13–17.

STUNKARD A. J. & PENICK S. B. (1979) Behaviour modification in the treatment of obesity: the problem of maintaining weight loss. *Archives of General Psychiatry* **36,** 801.

TAITZ L. F. (1971) Infantile overnutrition among artificially fed infants in the Sheffield region. *British Medical Journal* **1,** 315–16.

TANNER J. M. & WHITEHOUSE R. H. (1975) Revised standards for triceps and subscapular skinfolds in British children. *Archives of Disease in Childhood* **50,** 142.

TRACEY V. V., DE N. C. & HARPER J. R. (1971) Obesity and respiratory infections in infants and young children. *British Medical Journal* **1,** 16.

WILKINSON P. W., PARKIN J. M., PEARLSON G., STRONG H. & SYKES P. (1977) Energy intake and physical activity in obese chidren. Letter. *British Medical Journal* **1,** 756.

WHITEHEAD R. G., PAUL A. A. & COLE T. J. (1981) A critical analysis of measured food energy intakes during infancy and early childhood in comparison with current international recommendations. *Journal of Human Nutrition* **35,** 339–48.

WHITELAW A. G. L. (1971) The association of social class and sibling number with skinfold thickness in London schoolboys. *Human Biology* **43,** 414.

WHITELAW A. G. L. (1977) Infant feeding and subcutaneous fat at birth and at one year. *Lancet* **2,** 1098.

CHAPTER 3

Vitamins and Minerals

VITAMINS

A vitamin is an organic substance occuring in minute quantities in plant and animal tissues; it must be supplied in the diet or synthesized from essential dietary precursors. It is essential for specific metabolic functions to proceed normally. The nutritional role of vitamins, the consequence of deficiency and excess intake are dealt with in many nutrition books including those of Davidson *et al.* (1979) and McLaren & Burman (1982).

Factors Influencing Vitamin Utilization

A number of factors affect the availability of vitamins for their normal metabolic function:

1. **Availability in an absorbable form.** For example, niacin bound in maize is not available; fat-soluble vitamins are malabsorbed in steatorrhoea unless they are given in a water-miscible form.
2. **Anti-vitamins.** These compete with or inhibit the metabolic reaction in which the vitamin is involved or may be toxic of themselves, e.g., Avidin in uncooked egg white is an anti-vitamin to biotin.
3. **Pro-vitamins or precursors.** These must be converted into the active vitamin in the body, e.g., carotene is synthesized to vitamin A; tryptophan is converted to niacin; vitamin D is converted to 1,25-dihydroxycholecalciferol, the active form of the vitamin in the kidney, and failure of conversion largely accounts for the metabolic bone disease seen in patients with renal failure.
4. **Biosynthesis in the gut by intestinal flora.** Vitamin K, niacin, riboflavin, B_{12} and folic acid are synthesized by the bacterial flora of the intestine but they are relatively poorly

absorbed. Bacteria in the small intestine also use dietary vitamins and make requirements difficult to determine. Synthetic diets alter gut flora, also antibiotic therapy and infections change bacterial flora and therefore the synthesis of vitamins.

5. **Individual requirement.** Vitamin requirements, like all requirements, are a recommendation for the intake of a group of people as a whole and act only as a guide. Some individuals will vary in their requirement compared to the group. Catabolism increases requirements particularly of the water-soluble vitamins.

6. **Malabsorption.** Malabsorption increases vitamin needs and as a result particularly fat-soluble vitamin intake may need to be increased or supplied in water-miscible form. Specific diseases may increase the need for a specific vitamin, e.g., folate in untreated coeliac disease; vitamin E in cystic fibrosis and most dramatically in the rare condition abetalipoproteinaemia, where deficiency is present from birth and thereafter there are major defects in its absorption and transport (Muller *et al.* 1977).

7. **Competitors.** Some drugs compete with or neutralize vitamins and thus increase the requirement in the particular individual, e.g., di-iodohydroxyquinoline chelates calcium pantothenate and cholestyramine increases the need for folic acid.

8. **Amino acid imbalance.** An imbalance of amino acids can inhibit the uptake of amino acids and may lead to more severe vitamin deficiency, and raised amino acid levels may inhibit enzyme actions.

9. **Vitamin responsive metabolic disorders.** In a number of metabolic disorders involving an enzyme deficiency vitamin-responsive form of the disease occurs and responds to pharmaceutical doses of the specific co-enzyme vitamin involved, e.g.,

   (i)   Vitamin C in hawkinsonuria
  (ii) B_{12} in methylmalonic acidaemia
 (iii)   Thiamine in a rare variant of maple syrup urine disease
 (iv)   Pyridoxine is used to treat approximately 50% of cases with homocystinuria, and folic acid is a co-enzyme in another rare variant form of homocystinuria
  (v)   Ascorbic acid is used to reduce serum tyrosine levels in neonatal hypertyrosinaemia
 (vi)   Choline is a methyl donor in diets restricting the **sulphur amino acids cystine and methionine**

(vii) Folinic acid may be essential in a variant form of phenylketonuria related to pteridin metabolism.

As yet this is a relatively new area of research and it is probable that numerous other examples will be found in the next few years (See Francis in press).

10. **Inherited disorders of vitamin absorption.** A defect in intestinal absorption may be a major or a minor component of inherited disorders of vitamin absorption for example relating to B_{12} and folate (Chanarin 1982) and vitamin E (see 6. above).

Deficiency

With the exception of conditions related to vitamins D, E and K, diseases due to deficient intake of vitamins almost never occur in Britain in infants born at term.

Rickets and osteomalacia due to inadequate vitamin D intake still occur mainly in the Asian emigrant population (DHSS 1980a).

Familial hypophosphataemic rickets (vitamin D-resistant hypophosphataemic rickets) is a disorder of decreased renal tubular phosphate reabsorption with resultant bone demineralization, late-onset rickets, osteomalacia and growth retardation. Treatment is with inorganic phosphate and vitamin D ideally as 1,25-dihydroxycholecalciferol. The rickets seen in very low birth weight infants are most probably also related to phosphate deficiency rather than vitamin D deficiency alone (Hambidge & Walravens 1982).

Vitamin deficiencies are usually the result of insufficient vitamin intake, malabsorption such as cystic fibrosis, protracted diarrhoea and short gut syndrome, increased requirement, or the use of diets with a restricted intake of conventional food or enteral and elemental feeds, and synthetic diets without adequate supplementation. Rarely is one vitamin alone deficient (except for vitamin D) and where a recognizable deficiency is identified a severe lack of the vitamin can be assumed and may be in association with other vitamin deficiencies which are subclinical. Treatment with a comprehensive vitamin supplement is usually appropriate in order to prevent precipitation of other deficiencies.

In the developing world vitamin deficiencies are relatively common and vitamin A deficiency is a major cause of blindness in some areas.

Toxicity

Vitamin toxicity is mainly confined to the fat-soluble vitamins A and D. Excess water-soluble vitamins to the body's needs are either not absorbed and found in the faeces, or excreted in the urine.

The fashion of vitamin megaphagia is both wasteful and unnecessary. Harrell *et al.* (1981) suggested mega-vitamin supplementation in mentally retarded patients including those with Down's syndrome but others have shown these to be of no benefit (Smith *et al.* 1983). Long-term effects of mega-vitamin intakes need further evaluation before they can be regarded as either beneficial or indeed harmless.

ASCORBIC ACID

Briggs *et al.* (1973) have reported adverse effects of large doses of ascorbic acid which are metabolized to oxalate and excreted in urine. Oxalate stones may be produced with resultant damage to the kidney and bladder particularly in patients with an inborn ascorbic acid-induced hyperaloxuria (Briggs *et al.* 1973). However, doses of ascorbic acid in the magnitude of 1 g or more per day are only partially absorbed and oxalate formation remains approximately constant at levels about double the value found in subjects who are not receiving supplements (Hughes *et al.* 1981). The body adjusts to large doses of ascorbic acid and serum levels rise to a maximum about 9 days after regular supplementation, but then fall gradually and settle at a level which is not increased by larger doses. Sudden cessation of the large dose can lead to the development of scurvy on intakes that would normally be adequate (Rhead & Schrauzer 1971); infants have been reported to develop scurvy when preconditioned to high ascorbic acid intakes taken by the mother during pregnancy (Cochrane 1965).

An intake of 10 mg ascorbic acid per day can normally prevent scurvy; a generous intake of ascorbic acid may decrease the risk of heart disease and viral infections and therefore an intake in the range of 100 mg daily may be optimal but is preferably taken from natural fruit and vegetable sources which will simultaneously provide other nutrients such as potassium. A supplement of about 250 mg ascorbic acid for a few days at the first sign of an intercurrent infection may enhance recovery but long-term megadoses should be discouraged.

VITAMIN A

Acute poisoning occurs occasionally in hypersensitive individuals even from a single excessive dose (100 000 µg). Symptoms include restlessness, headache and vomiting with raised intercranial pressure (McLaren 1982). Treatment is to stop vitamin A supplements. Chronic poisoning takes several weeks to occur and has been reported due to doses in the range of 20 000 µg per day. A fasting plasma vitamin A level of 250 µg/100 ml or more is diagnostic. Symptoms of the chronic vitamin A poisoning are non-specific including hair changes, dry rough skin, cracked lips.

Carotenaemia which is probably harmless is characterized by yellow pigmentation of the palms and is associated with excess intake of carrots, apricots and other high carotene foods. It is most freqently seen in young children, and some adolescents with anorexia nervosa, taking large quantities of fruit and vegetables. The increased use of 'health foods', vitamin supplements and carrot juice or apricots necessitates an awareness of such conditions which may be overlooked or incorrectly diagnosed unless a careful dietary history is taken. Treatment is by withdrawal of vitamin A supplements and a reduction of carotene intake to normal levels.

VITAMIN D

A relatively small excess of vitamin D equivalent to about 30 to 100 µg per day has been associated with hypercalcaemia. However hypercalcaemia due to excess vitamin D is relatively uncommon compared to the 1950s when infant formulae were overfortified. Since then the permitted fortification has been reduced and better controlled (DHSS 1980a). As many proprietary vitamin supplements can be obtained care should be taken that only one supplement is given at any time and the correct dose is given (DHSS 1980a).

The use of the active form of vitamin D as 1,25-cholecalciferol in the treatment of the bone disease associated with chronic renal disease requires careful monitoring of the dose and any hypercalcaemia that occurs must be treated with a reduction of the supplement and a temporary reduced intake of dietary calcium and supplements. A small number of patients will acquire hypercalcaemia due to idiopathic hypercalcaemia; such patients may be particularly sensitive to vitamin D.

Vitamins in Normal Nutrition

Human milk provides the infant with adequate nutrition for the first months of life. A healthy mother who has had a nutritionally adequate diet and who has been exposed to sunlight will be able to supply her baby with a milk which contains all the vitamins known to be necessary, and vitamin deficiencies are not normally seen. Vitamin D sulphate has been found in the aqueous fraction of human milk in the range of 2 µg per 100 ml in early lactation decreasing to 0.8 µg per 100 ml in mature milk, whereas the fat-soluble vitamin D content is only 0.01 µg per 100 ml (DHSS 1980b). This may account for the clinical observation that rickets are uncommon in breast-fed infants. However, vitamin D deficiency does still occur, chiefly amongst low birth weight infants and those born to Asian emigrants to Britain. The importance of vitamin D supplements in these groups cannot be over emphasized (DHSS 1980a) in order to reduce the prevalence of fetal and infantile rickets and osteomalacia in older children.

Proprietary infant formulae which meet the recommended compositional guidelines (DHSS 1980b) contain added vitamins. When mixed feeding is introduced and particularly once the infant changes to cow's milk, there is a greater risk of vitamin D deficiency, particularly if there is insufficient exposure to sunlight on the bare skin for adequate vitamin D synthesis. Most household diets are adequate in other vitamins. However, there are some infants offered a diet which contains inadequate vitamins and other infants are reluctant to eat a variety of vitamin-containing conventional foods. A supplement of vitamins A, D and C is therefore recommended from the time the child is 1 month old and should continue until at least 2 years and preferably 5 years old. The standard 5 drops per day dose of Children's Vitamin A, D, C, Drops contains 200 µg vitamin A, 20 mg vitamin C and 7.5 µg vitamin D. This provides a safe dose of vitamins even when used in conjunction with fortified milk formulae except for the very rare case of a patient with idiopathic hypercalcaemia. The equivalent amount of vitamin D can be given from other proprietary vitamin supplements (Table 3.1) but more than one supplement must be avoided. If there is no doubt that the diet of an individual is adequate, supplements can be omitted.

For the older child the other vitamins are plentifully supplied by a mixed diet including human or cow's milk, cereals, fruits, vegetables, meat, eggs, butter or margarine, and are not normally required as supplements. However, goat's milk is low in folic acid and vitamin B_{12}, and both cow's milk and goat's milk are low in available iron. Young children having goat's milk in place of cow's milk, in addition to vitamins A, D and C, should have a source of folic acid and vitamin B_{12} as well as iron from conventional foods or supplements. Anaemia can occur when children are given these milks as the major source of nutrition without supplements.

Vegans and vegetarians are recommended vitamin B_{12} supplements, as non-carnivorous foods do not contain this vitamin and although the intestinal flora provide some vitamin B_{12}, the intake is variable and unreliable.

Preterm and low birth weight infants have increased requirements for vitamins including vitamin D.

Vitamins in Therapeutic Diets

The artificial nature of many therapeutic diets will inevitably mean that certain essential vitamins will not be available from food and these must, therefore, be provided in an acceptable alternative form. When substituting normal food with man-made products or where great restriction of natural foods exists, it is important that the lesser known nutrients are not overlooked. It has been shown that rashes, and failure to thrive, can result from deficiency of such vitamins as choline chloride, calcium pantothenate, vitamin K, inositol, biotin, vitamin E, vitamin B_{12} and folic acid (Mann *et al.* 1965). These vitamins are frequently not present in multivitamin supplements and may not be added to enteral feeds, elemental diets and milk substitutes used in therapeutic diets (Tripp *et al.* 1974; Bunker & Clayton 1983) or parenteral nutrition regimens. The diets used for milk and disaccharide intolerance, galactosaemia, phenylketonuria, amino acid disorders, in restricted diets such as are used in renal failure and in patients with malabsorption, or with multiple food allergy, should be provided with a complete range of vitamins supplied either in the milk substitute or separately as a comprehensive vitamin supplement (Tables 3.1 and 3.2) such as Ketovites (Paines & Byrne) or Cow & Gate Vitamin-Mineral Supplement Tablets. Forceval Junior Capsules (Unigreg) and the Seravit preparations (SHS) have the advantage of a single dose to provide a variety of vitamins and some minerals (Table 3.2). The Ketovite preparations (Table 3.1) contain adequate amounts of all known vitamins required by man. Both tablets and liquid are required, the one not being a substitute for the other, as the tablets contain the 11 water-soluble vitamins and the supplement liquid contains vitamins A, D, B_{12} and choline chloride in a water-miscible carbohydrate-free base. As they are free of carbohydrate, sorbitol and colouring, they are suitable for

Table 3.1 Comparison of various vitamin supplements with human and cow's milk (normal recommended full dose of vitamin supplements). (Data from manufacturers 1984).

Vitamin		Human milk mature 100 ml	Pasteurized cow's milk 100 ml	Children's Vitamin A, D, C, Drops (Welfare Food Supplies) 5 drops	Adexolin drops (Farley) 7 drops	Abidec drops (Parke Davis) 0.6 ml
Vitamin A	μg	60.0	Av. 33.4 + Carotene	200.0	315	1200.0
Thiamine B_1	mg	0.02	0.04	Nil	Nil	1.0
Riboflavin B_2	mg	0.03	0.19	Nil	Nil	0.4
Vitamin B_{12}	μg	Trace	0.3	Nil	Nil	Nil
Ascorbic acid C	mg	3.7	1.5	20.0	21	50.0
Retinol D	μg	0.025	0.02	7.5	7	10.0
Nicotinic acid/ Niacin	mg	0.22	0.08	Nil	Nil	5.0
Pantothenic acid	mg	0.25	0.35	Nil	Nil	Nil
Pyridoxine B_6	mg	0.01	0.04	Nil	Nil	0.5
Vitamin E	mg	0.34	0.09	Nil	Nil	Nil
Biotin	μg	0.7	2.0	Nil	Nil	Nil
Folic acid (total)	μg	5.0	5.0	Nil	Nil	Nil
Inositol	mg	N/S	N/S	Nil	Nil	Nil
Choline	mg	N/S	N/S	Nil	Nil	Nil
Vitamin K	mg	Trace	Trace	Nil	Nil	Nil

[a] For intravenous infusion and use with parenteral nutrition

[b] In intra-lipid. Present in unspecified quantity.

N/S not specified.

most patients with various intolerances. The Cow & Gate Vitamin-Mineral Supplement Tablets (Table 3.2) are adequate if used in conjunction with a vitamin A and D preparation, or Ketovite liquid. They contain 70 mg sucrose per tablet as the filler and are, therefore, unsuitable where traces of carbohydrate are significant, e.g., fructosaemia; but are usually tolerated by patients with secondary disaccharide intolerance. They contain some trace minerals and iron in addition to vitamins. The tablets can be crushed and added to an infant's feed immediately prior to giving it, provided that the infant will consume all the feed. However,

Dalivit drops (Paines & Byrne)	Paladac multi-vitamin supplement (Parke Davis)	Ketovite (Paines & Byrne) 3 tablets + 5 ml liquid	MVI Multi-vitamin[a] (SAS)	Solivito[a] (Kabivitrum)	Vita-lipid[a] Infant (Kabivitrum)
0.6 ml	5 ml	liquid	3 ml	1 vial	1 ml
1500.0	1200	750.0	900.0	Nil	100.0
1.0	3	3.0	15.0	1.2	Nil
0.4	3	3.0	3.0	1.8	Nil
Nil	Nil	12.5	Nil	2.0	Nil
50.0	50	50.0	150.0	30.0	Nil
10.0	10	10.0	7.5	Nil	2.5
5.0	20	10.0	30.0	10.0	Nil
Nil	Nil	3.5	7.5	10.0	Nil
0.5	1	1.0	4.5	2.0	Nil
Nil	Nil	15.0	1.5 iu	Nil	b
Nil	Nil	500.0	Nil	300.0	Nil
Nil	Nil	750.0	Nil	200.0	Nil
Nil	Nil	150.0	Nil	Nil	Nil
Nil	Nil	150.0	Nil	Nil	Nil
Nil	Nil	1.5	Nil	Nil	0.5

vitamin supplements should normally be given as a medicine and not added to infant feeds. The first year of life is the most critical for growth and development and the requirement of vitamins is higher due to the rapid synthesis of tissue. Comprehensive vitamin supplements should be given and continued at least in the pre-school child unless the intake of conventional food provides an adequate range and quantity of vitamins, and for so long as the therapeutic diet is continued in conjunction with very restricted diets, irrespective of age. Specific (co-enzyme) vitamins used to treat vitamin-responsive metabolic and inherited vitamin disorders must be continued for the lifetime.

Table 3.2 Comparison of various vitamin-mineral supplements. (Data from manufacturers 1984).

		Cow & Gate Vitamin-Mineral Supplement Tablets	Forceval Capsules (Unigreg)	Scientific Hospital Supplies		
				Seravit (Adult)	Modified Seravit (079)	Infant Seravit (222)
		Each tablet	Each capsule	100 g	100 g	100 g
Vitamin A	μg	Nil	1500	6500	3200	8325
Thiamine B$_1$	mg	0.25	10	11.6	5.8	6.25
Riboflavin B$_2$	mg	0.25	5	11.6	5.8	9.37
Vitamin B$_{12}$	μg	1.0	2	36	18	15.0
Ascorbic acid C	mg	10	50	566	283	640.6
Retinol D	μg	Nil	15	38	19.0	117.5
Nicotinic acid/Niacin	mg	0.8	20	83.2	41.6	70.3
Pantothenic acid	mg	0.5[a]	2[a]	36.6	20	27.3
Pyridoxine B$_6$	mg	0.08	0.5	15	7.5	5.4
Tocopherol E	mg	1.24	10	166	83	77.3
Biotin	μg	8	N/S	1160	583	400
Folic acid (total)	μg	63	N/S	1660	833	600
Inositol	mg	N/S	60	184	92	1562.5
Choline	mg	N/S	40	1832	916	1015.6
Vitamin K	mg	0.125	N/S	3.92	1.96	0.7
l-Lysine	mg	Nil	60	Nil	Nil	Nil
Calcium	mmol	N/S	1.75	N/S	100	112.5
Potassium	mmol	N/S	0.08	N/S	102.6	N/S
Sodium	mmol	N/S	N/S	N/S	108.7	N/S

Magnesium	mmol	N/S	0.08	51.4	25.7	25.7
Chloride	mmol	N/S	N/S	N/S	114.1	N/S
Phosphorus	mmol	N/S	1.8	51.6	129	96.8
Iron	mmol	0.015	0.18	1.5	0.75	1.8
Copper	μmol	0.53	7.9	129	65.0	118
Zinc	μmol	9.5	7.7	1272	636	1100
Manganese	μmol	0.09	9.1	226	113	132
Iodine	μmol	0.09	0.8	5.3	2.6	6
Molybdenum	μmol	0.06	N/S	6.9	3.47	5
Aluminium	μmol	N/S	N/S	0.32	0.16	N/S
Chromium	μmol	N/S	N/S	1.7	0.87	5
Selenium	μmol	N/S	N/S	N/S	N/S	4
Carbohydrate	g	0.07[b]	Nil	88[c]	62[c]	65[c]
Normal dose per day		6 to 12 tablets	1 capsule	25 g[d]	20 g	8 to 12 g

[a] As calcium pantothenate.
[b] Sucrose.
[c] Maltodextrin.
[d] If used for children the appropriate dose must be calculated.
N/s not specified.

MINERALS

A mineral is considered nutritionally essential when an animal species deprived of it develops reproducible features which can be prevented or reversed by supplementation with physiological amounts of that mineral. A number of minerals including those required in so-called trace quantities are necessary for normal nutrition. The essential minerals for man include calcium, phosphorus, sulphur, magnesium, sodium, potassium, chlorine, iron, zinc, copper, manganese, iodine, cobalt, molybdenum, chromium, selenium; others such as nickel, fluorine, tin, vanadium, silicon and arsenic have been reported essential in other mammals but direct evidence of a nutritional requirement in man is awaited (Davies 1981; Aggett & Davies 1983). Virtually every inorganic mineral is found in human tissue including the heavy metals, lead, mercury, cadmium and strontium. Any mineral in excess quantity may be toxic (Underwood 1977) but this is especially true of the heavy metals, e.g., cadmium, lead and mercury. The nutritional requirement for the macro minerals calcium, phosphorus (Table 1.2), sulphur, magnesium, sodium, potassium and chlorine are well established and data of their content in foods is available. The biological function of these macro minerals is well documented (Underwood 1977; Davidson *et al.* 1979; McLaren & Burman 1982). However, the role of the trace minerals is still not clearly understood; knowledge of the available content in food is often unsatisfactory or of only limited use and nutritional requirements in health and disease are still not clearly established. There is now a rapidly growing accumulation of data regarding the nutritional importance of the trace minerals including their biological function, deficiency states and factors affecting their interactions and bioavailability (WHO 1973; Underwood 1977). The trace element symposium issue of the *Journal of Inherited Metabolic Disease* Vol. 6, No. 1, 1983, is a particularly useful reference source of information and the Nestlé 8th Nutrition Workshop on *Trace Minerals* which is due to be published in 1986.

The trace minerals are the inorganic equivalent of the vitamins, and as they cannot be synthesized by organisms, must be present in the diet. Their essential biological role is in their indispensibility to a large number of enzyme activities either as an integral part of the enzyme-protein molecules or as an activator of the enzyme, for example zinc is essential for the alkaline phosphatase, carbonic anhydrase and alcohol dehydrogenase, and copper for cytochrome oxidase and tyrosinase. This is not always the case and some metals, e.g., zinc regulate metabolic processes such as cell division and growth by as yet undefined mechanisms. They are involved in the synthesis of protein, DNA and RNA. Zinc is needed for wound healing and growth; chromium is needed for carbohydrate metabolism and copper is essential for adequate utilization of iron.

Knowledge of the trace minerals content of food has been largely unsatisfactory until recently because of inaccuracies inherent in the older analytical methods; noncomparability between different studies due to sampling techniques and analytical method differences, imprecise identification of the food, its origin, variety, processing and preparation. There are also major regional differences in the content of the minerals in food grown in different areas as illustrated by the incidence of endemic goitre in places where there are low levels of iodine in soil, water and food (Underwood 1977) and the different regions within a country such as food grown in the selenium-deficient soils of New Zealand and China (Underwood 1977).

The dietary intake of minerals are greatly influenced by the choice of foods consumed and by their origin. For example, individuals on low income diets are at particular risk from marginal or inadequate zinc intake because the best dietary sources of the mineral are often the more expensive foods, especially meat.

Factors Influencing Mineral Utilization

Physico-chemical Properties
Physico-chemical properties and the co-ordination compounds formed with other dietary constituents and products of intraluminal hydrolysis influence the mucosal uptake of the trace minerals (Forth & Rummel 1975). Such compounds may for example enhance uptake by maintaining the mineral in a water-soluble form.

Phosphate
Phosphate from food or its processing reduces the bioavailability of iron, zinc and copper as do the major organic phosphate dietary compounds, phytate and casein.
    1. Phytate (myo-Inositol 1,2,3,4,5,6-hexakis dihydrogen phosphate) is a compound which occurs naturally in many foods

derived from plants including all cereals, many legumes including soya, nuts, some fruit, tubers and roots. Phytate has been recognized as a nutrient, because it contains phosphorus, but it is also considered toxic because it binds various essential minerals and reduces their availability for absorption from the diet and reabsorption after their secretion in digestive juices (Wise 1983). The complex interactions of phytate with dietary components in the gut have been recently reviewed by Wise (1983) who develops the theory that:

'. . . the prime factor determining the fate of phytate in the intestine is the ratio of calcium to phytate. In the absence of calcium, the concentration of trace metals may be insufficient to precipitate phytate which then may be hydrolysed by mucosal phytase, but the activity of this enzyme will depend on the presence of zinc and vitamin D. When the amount of calcium present is insufficient to precipitate all the phytate, very small particles are precipitated and a proportion of the trace metals studied bind to this complex, whereas the rest remain in solution. Some phytate may be hydrolysed by phytase. When there is sufficient calcium to precipitate all the phytate, the complex is poorly available to mucosal phytase and practically all of the trace metals studied bind to the complex. However, a high proportion of the trace metals are accessible for desorption by amino acids, and excess calcium competes for binding sites with cadmium. Therefore, increased dietary protein and calcium would lead to greater desorption in the small intestine. When the calcium phytate reaches the caecum, it may be hydrolysed by bacteria and the calcium released for absorption, though trace metals may remain bound to the unhydrolysed complex. A high concentration of calcium decreases the activity of microbial phytase, and it is possible that dietary fibre components might modify activity of microbial phytase.'

It is possible that the protein-calcium-phytate complexes are favoured in the presence of low calcium concentrations and that these have greater solubility than calcium phytate. Calcium deficiency rarely occurs when there is a low calcium to phytate ratio according to Walker (1951) from his world-wide survey into human high phytate diets.

Different plant sources of phytate influence zinc availability to different extents (Franz *et al.* 1980). Zinc in soya bean is apparently not associated with phytate, but once it reaches the intestine, the phytate decreases the availability of the zinc (Ellis

& Morris 1981) but not that of calcium (Erdman 1979), possibly because the calcium phytate carries a considerable proportion of the dietary zinc past the major sites of absorption in the small intestine, whereas the calcium is subsequently released by bacteria and absorbed in the colon. Any zinc released by the hydrolysis of other particles would be bound by any remaining unhydrolyzed calcium phytate thus inhibiting zinc absorption even if the colon were able to absorb some zinc (Wise 1983). The detrimental effect of dietary phytate on zinc absorption can be reduced by increased dietary protein (Davies 1982).

Increasing intakes of calcium further reduces zinc availability by lowering the zinc to phytate molar ratio needed to induce zinc deficiency in rats receiving otherwise physiological intakes of zinc (Davies 1982). The present traditional diet in the UK has been calculated to have a zinc to phytate molar ratio of 1:6 to 1:8 and the calcium intake needed to seriously impair zinc availability would be 3 to 7 g daily which is in excess of our usual intake (Aggett & Davies 1983).

Negative zinc balances in man have been reported with zinc to phytate molar ratios of 1:10 to 1:13 (Aggett & Davies 1983).

The recent recommendations (James 1983) to decrease the national diet's fat intake and to increase dietary fibre will inevitably result in an increased phytate intake due to increased use of cereals, fruit and vegetables. A reduced zinc intake may also occur due to a decreased use of meat in the diet. In addition if the fibre intake is increased by enhancing refined cereals with bran, a further reduction in zinc could occur. As a result of these changes the zinc to phytate molar ratio could fall into the range of 1:10 or more and negative zinc balance could occur, at least in some individuals. Textured vegetable proteins have been found to have a zinc to phytate molar ratio of more than 1:25 and hence are not recommended as a total replacement of meat, and in some vegan diets a zinc to phytate molar ratio of 1:244 has been reported by Harland & Petersen (1978).

Phytase in yeast will reduce the mineral binding capacity of the phytate in flour during fermentation. Dephytenized bran products are now becoming available (Andersson *et al.* 1983).

2.   The phospho-protein casein. This binds zinc which is only released at a pH below 4.6. The variable gastric acid secretion and pancreatic proteolytic function in neonates may make them vulnerable to reduced bioavailability of zinc induced by casein (Harzer & Kauer 1982). This has yet to be confirmed *in* *vivo* but it may partly account for the low zinc availability from cow's milk which has sufficient casein to bind all the zinc present. Human milk with its lower casein content has more zinc associated with low molecular weight ligands which may facilitate its absorption (Harzer & Kauer 1982). Two ligands, picolinic acid and citric acid, which prevent the zinc casein complex formation *in vitro* are destroyed in processing of formulae based on cow's milk and therefore may reduce zinc availability; of these only citrate has been unequivocally identified in human breast milk.

Fibre

Reinhold *et al.* (1976) suggested that fibre may reduce the bioavailability of trace minerals and the effect may be additive to that of phytate. Fibre does increase faecal output and there is a trend towards a decrease in transit time with a high fibre intake. However, recent work by Andersson *et al.* (1983) indicates that wheat-bran, and in particular the cell-wall polysaccharides of bran in amounts customarily eaten, are unlikely to exert a significant effect on mineral absorption in man, independently of the effect of the phytate present in bran. The reduced bioavailability of minerals observed with high fibre diets is related to their phytate content with the possible exception of iron retention which in Andersson and his colleague's study (1983) showed a tendency to decrease with increasing amounts of bran in the diet. They suggest that there is some substance in bran, besides phytic acid, which may have a slight negative effect on iron absorption. Individuals transferring from white to wholemeal bread and adding raw bran and All-bran to their diets had a negative calcium balance over a 3-week period in the study by Cummings *et al.* (1979), but this is now identified by Andersson *et al.* (1983) as being due to the effect of the increased phytate content of the dietary change.

The importance of identifying the phytate in bran as the major cause of mineral malabsorption lies in the widespread use of unprocessed bran and high fibre diets. To avoid the dangers of mineral imbalance raw bran should be avoided. A better source of fibre is food such as wholemeal bread where the action of phytase in yeast will have reduced the mineral-binding capacity of the phytate very considerably during fermentation. Alternatively, the dephytenized bran products which are now becoming available (if necessary) should be used (Andersson *et al.* 1983), or the lower phytate cereals such as oats can be used more extensively in the diet.

Animal Protein

Animal protein such as egg, milk, beef, cheese, and casein significantly increases the bioavailability of zinc from wholemeal bread which is high in phytate. Thus, the adverse effect may be minimized by a mixed diet.

Trace Mineral Interactions

Minerals of similar physico-chemical properties may antagonize one another, e.g., copper deficiency can be precipitated by a physiological or high zinc intake in rats on marginally inadequate copper intakes; the reverse occurs in pigs who become zinc-deficient on high copper intakes. Zinc supplements in human patients with both sickle cell anaemia and coeliac disease have been associated with hypocupraemia, anaemia and neutropenia as a result of copper deficiency (Aggett & Davies 1983). A corollary of this is the use of oral zinc supplements in the management of Wilson's disease in which copper is handled abnormally (Van Caillie-Bertrand *et al.* 1985).

Interactions have been observed in animals and reviewed by Forth & Rummel (1975) e.g., rats and mice with iron deficiency have enhanced uptake of cobalt, manganese, zinc, iron, cadmium and lead; zinc, cobalt, chromium and iron uptakes are improved in zinc-deficient rats. The significance of these findings for human nutrition is not known but these and other interactions should be borne in mind when planning dietary supplementation and trace element therapy (Aggett & Davies 1983) and there should be a critical and practical evaluation of the level of trace elements provided by different diets and formulae. This is particularly important when considering infant formulae, synthetic and therapeutic diets, enteral feeds and parenteral nutrition. For example, the iron:zinc molar ratio of different infant formulae has been reviewed by Aggett & Davies (1983). The ratio in human and cow's milk is approximately 0.4 whereas formulae vary between Ostermilk 5.3, Prosobee 2.8, Wysoy 2.2, and Gold Cap SMA 2.1 which may not be optimal for the utilization of these minerals (Aggett & Davies 1983).

Evaluation of Trace Mineral Intakes

An evaluation, by trace mineral balance, of a home-made trace element supplement used with Galactomin (Cow & Gate) highlights the difficulties encountered in devising supplements on theoretical grounds alone (Aggett *et al.* 1983). The authors proposed the high iron content of the supplement as a possible cause of the poor retention of the zinc and copper in these infants. The theoretical intake of trace minerals required to achieve a net retention comparable to those seen in the healthy children would likewise not be fully met by the Cow & Gate Vitamin-Mineral Supplement Tablets (Table 3.2) originally for use with Galactomin, manganese and copper being inadequate (Aggett *et al.* 1983). The zinc content of the home-made trace element supplement has been subsequently increased (see Table 3.7 for the current formula) since this work was carried out, and before publication of the results.

Metabolic balance studies to evaluate a comprehensive mineral mixture (I) used in the treatment of children with phenylketonuria (Alexander *et al.* 1974) showed the zinc and manganese intakes were less than those of healthy children and copper and iron were inadequate to maintain a positive balance. An amended formula (II) was evaluated by Lawson *et al.* (1977) and was found satisfactory for synthetic diets based on amino acids. This amended formula (II) is currently available as Aminogran Mineral Mixture (Allen & Hanbury Ltd.) (see Table 3.6). When Thorn and her colleagues (1978) evaluated these same two comprehensive mineral mixtures in infants receiving the Comminuted Chicken-based module formula for the management of protracted diarrhoea, she found the infants on the comprehensive mineral mixture (I) to be in negative zinc balance despite a higher intake of zinc that that of healthy children; those on the comprehensive mineral mixture (II) were in positive zinc balance and this formula has been used extensively in this and similar regimens subsequently. In retrospect Aggett & Davies (1983) suggest the reason for the reduced bioavailability of the zinc in the infants on the mineral mixture formula I in conjunction with an animal-based protein (Comminuted Chicken), may be related to the iron supplementation these infants were receiving before or during the balance studies. These formulae do not contain chromium or selenium. Lombeck *et al.* (1984) have made recommendations for selenium intakes for patients receiving treatment with synthetic diets for conditions such as phenylketonuria.

Deficiency

Precise deficiency states have been associated with a number of the trace minerals (Table 3.3). Although it is relatively easy to confirm

Table 3.3 Clinical presentation of various trace mineral deficiencies.

Mineral	Feature	Reference
Chromium	Impaired glucose tolerance; Lipid disorders	Saner 1980, Aggett & Davies 1983
	Encephalopathy, neuropathy	
	In conjunction with parenteral nutrition	
		Jeejeebhoy *et al.* 1977, Freund *et al.* 1979, *Lancet*, Editorial 1983
Copper	Bone lesions; Connective tissue disorders; Neutropenia; Anaemia; Diarrhoea in infants	Camakaris *et al.* 1983
	In conjunction with parenteral nutrition	Karpel & Pedan 1972
Manganese	Impaired gluconeogensis	Aggett & Davies 1983
	Weight loss or impaired growth; Hypocholesterolaemia; Prolonged prothrombin time	Doisey 1972[a]
Molybdenum	None observed under natural conditions	
	Reduced growth;[b] Impaired uric acid metabolism[b]	Coughlan 1983, Wadman 1983
	In conjunction with parenteral nutrition	Abumrad *et al.* 1981
Selenium	Muscle pain and weakness; Poor growth in children or synthetic diets; Poor growth in children with kwashiorkor In conjunction with parenteral nutrition	Lombeck 1983, Lombeck 1984, Fleming *et al.* 1982 *Lancet*, Editorial 1983
Zinc	Growth retardation Skin rashes; Hair loss; Anorexia; Poor wound healing; Impaired taste and smell; Reduced immune response; Diarrhoea	Vallee 1983, Aggett & Harries 1979, Aggett 1983, Aggett & Davies 1983
	In conjunction with parenteral nutrition	Kay *et al.* 1976

[a] Only in one reported case in association with Vitamin K deficiency.
[b] In experimental animals.

deficiencies associated with severe malnutrition marginal deficiencies are more difficult to detect and evaluation by dietary survey and calculated intakes are inadequate due to the varying bioavailability and interaction of the minerals; clinical and laboratory criteria provide some indication and may only be confirmed in retrospect following correction of a defect following supplementation.

A number of situations predispose an individual to a potential or actual deficiency of trace minerals (Table 3.4). The most vulnerable are individuals with protein-energy malnutrition, and those with increased metabolic demands due to growth in infants and children, pregnancy, lactation and catabolic states, also those on synthetic diets and parenteral nutrition (Aggett & Davies 1983; *Lancet*, Editorial 1983). Malabsorption also predisposes to mineral deficiencies.

The risk of developing deficiency will also depend on body reserves. Although there are no specific reserves of zinc in the body it can be released from bone or muscle at times of deprivation or catabolism and thus plasma levels may not fall and symptomatic deficiency may be averted (Fell *et al.* 1973). However, growth may be limited by zinc supply during renutrition of malnourished children, with a consequent fall in plasma zinc (Golden & Golden 1981). Thus, the zinc requirement, the plasma zinc concentration and the likelihood of symptomatic deficiency are dependent on whether the subject is in an anabolic or catabolic state. Specific reserves of copper and iron cushion the impact of their deprivation. In the preterm infant such reserves have not accumulated and the high growth rate and inefficient absorption of trace minerals predisposes these infants to deficiency (Mendelson *et al.* 1983). There appear to be no body reserves of manganese and it is as yet unknown if stores of chromium, selenium or molybdenum exist.

The balance studies recently conducted by Mendelson and colleagues (1983) showed preterm infants fed their own mother's fresh milk received copper and zinc but not iron in recommended amounts. These infants achieved estimated *in utero* retention rates for copper at each age studied and achieved the estimated *in vitro* retention rate for zinc at 4 weeks, but they retained insufficient iron throughout the study. In comparison the infants fed a formula SMA 24 (J. Wyeth USA) received all 3 minerals in the recommended quantities but the apparent copper and iron retentions were below that expected *in utero*. Mendelson *et al.* concluded that despite the high bioavailability of iron from preterm human milk, adequate retention could not be achieved even if absorption was complete.

Table 3.4 Conditions predisposing to a risk of trace mineral deficiency in man. (Adapted from Aggett & Davies 1983.)

---

1 Inadequate dietary intake and/or bioavailability
Preterm infants
Protein-energy malnutrition
Restricted protein intake
Synthetic and therapeutic diets, e.g. for management of inborn errors of metabolism or malabsorption states
Low socio-economic income groups
High fibre and phytate diets particularly in association with low animal protein intake
Replacement of meat intake solely with vegetable textured proteins
Vegetarian, vegan diets and cult diets, e.g. Zen macrobiotic diets, fruitarian diets
Parenteral nutrition
Formulae and enternal feeds as the sole source of nutrition

2 Malabsorption
Immaturity of absorptive mechanisms
Intestinal enteropathies, e.g. coeliac disease, cow's milk protein intolerance
Pancreatic insufficiency
Short gut syndrome
Inborn errors of mineral absorption; acrodermatitis enteropathica; Menke's disease
Achlorhydria

3 Increased body losses
Catabolic states, e.g. starvation, burns, infection
Diabetes mellitus
Diuretic therapy, proteinuria (Nephrotic syndrome), hepatic disease, dialysis
Chronic blood loss
Skin diseases, e.g. eczema, acrodermatitis bullosa
Protein-losing enteropathies
Excessive sweating in the case of zinc
Intravascular haemolysis, porphyria
Chelating agent therapy

The iron from the fortified formula was poorly absorbed. Also high doses of iron reduce zinc and copper absorption as well as counteracting the beneficial role of the lactoferrin in human milk. It is therefore suggested that iron supplements should be delayed until the preterm infant's iron stores are exhausted at about 6 to 8 weeks which corresponds to the increase in the rate of erythrocyte formation, when the infant is more likely to benefit from iron supplements (Mendelson *et al.* 1983). The zinc and copper content of preterm human milk is greater than that of mature human milk and these minerals appear to be better retained by the infant if the milk is fed fresh, that is, neither pasteurized nor frozen which, for example, may modify the effectiveness of some zinc binding compounds, thus reducing the zinc availability. Even so, preterm fresh human milk may not always fully protect these infants from zinc deficiency if the intake of milk is low (Aggett *et al.* 1980) or if there is a defect in the mammary zinc secretion (Zimmerman *et al.* 1982). Whether the newer preterm and low birth weight formulae are more appropriate in zinc, copper and iron remains to be established.

Zinc and some other trace minerals are bound to milk proteins (Harzer & Kauer 1982) and are therefore partly removed during the manufacture of modified infant milk because of their lower protein content. Also the whey used is demineralized to remove excess calcium, sodium and potassium which further reduces the inorganic zinc and other minerals which are replaced with organic supplements. Organic supplements are often less well absorbed than their inorganic counterparts and therefore trace mineral deficiencies may result from otherwise desirable modifications of milk for infant feeding. The guidelines for the composition of artificial feeds based on cow's milk for the young infant (DHSS 1980b) do not include figures for trace minerals apart from iron. The Joint FAO/WHO Food Standards Programme Codex Alimentarius Commission (FAO/WHO 1976) included recommended levels for magnesium, iron, iodine, copper, zinc and manganese. The WHO Trace Elements in Human Nutrition Committee (1973) recommends that such formulae should contain all essential trace minerals including, in addition to those given by the Codex Alimentarius Committee, chromium, vanadium, nickel, tin and selenium at least to the levels present in human milk. However, as can be seen from the work on bioavailability and retention of minerals already discussed, evaluation other than compositional comparison is essential. The increasing use of soya-isolate formulae (up to 25% of the infants fed on artificial formulae in the USA) necessitates further evaluation for trace mineral availability, particularly in the light of their phytate content which can inhibit the availability of zinc, calcium and iron (O'Dell 1979; Aggett & Davies 1983). It is not feasible to predict the availability and therefore the appropriate content of trace minerals in diets and formulae based on soya, amino acids, or hydrolyzed proteins.

Recommended Intakes

Requirements for the macro minerals are discussed in Chapter 1 and summarized in Table 1.2. As yet no recommended intakes or actual requirements have been set in the UK for trace minerals. A WHO Trace Elements in Human Nutrition Committee (1973) and the National Research Council (1980) have published recommended intakes to cover normal physiological needs for trace minerals. Allowances for increased needs during illness have not been considered. Aggett & Davies (1983) have summarized these recommendations and estimated safe and adequate intakes (Table 3.5) which tend to be generous, and do not take into account any increased efficiency of absorption that may occur with low intakes. The adequacy of a dietary intake cannot be determined by the calculated trace mineral content alone as the availability for absorption is critical and the bioavailability especially of iron and zinc varies with the type of diet. Supplements can cause an imbalance and may actually worsen the overall trace mineral status. It is therefore essential to use these recommended intakes as a presumed adequate range and not as an index for the determination of suboptimal nutrition in an individual.

Minerals in Normal Nutrition

A well-balanced mixed diet of conventional foods which provides adequate amounts of the other nutrient requirements is most likely to provide an adequate intake of trace minerals. The increased use of refined carbohydrates and fat in the Western diet has reduced the intake of trace minerals; white flour has a lower trace mineral content than wholemeal, sugar has negligible content and modern packaging and processing has largely eliminated food contamination which in the past no doubt provided a source of some trace minerals.

Infants should be breast-fed whenever possible. Colostrum and human milk are excellent sources of trace minerals including iron in a biologically available form (McMillan *et al.* 1976; Mendelson *et al.* 1983).

The nutritional requirements of trace minerals like those of other nutrients are less well known for the preterm and low birth weight infant whose stores of certain nutrients are lower than those of the normal infant, and in whom mucosal absorption may be impaired. The absorption and retention of copper and zinc was considered to be suboptimal in low birth weight infants fed pasteurized pooled breast milk, fortified with ferrous sulphate and vitamins A, D and C (Dauncey *et al.* 1977). A recent study compared the mineral content of preterm and full-term human milk and found higher

Table 3.5 Recommended dietary allowances (iron and zinc) and estimated safe and adequate intakes of other trace metals per day. (Adapted from Aggett & Davies 1983 and NRC 1980).

Age	Iron mmol	Zinc μmol	Copper μmol	Manganese μmol	Chromium μmol	Selenium μmol	Molybdenum μmol
0 to 6 months	0.18	46	7.8 to 11.0	9.1 to 12.8	0.19 to 0.77	0.13 to 0.5	0.31 to 0.63
6 to 12 months	0.18	76	11.0 to 16.0	12.8 to 18.2	0.38 to 1.15	0.25 to 0.76	0.41 to 0.83
1 to 3 years	0.27	153	16.0 to 23.6	18.2 to 27.3	0.38 to 1.5	0.25 to 1.01	0.52 to 1.0
4 to 6 years	0.18	153	23.6 to 31.5	27.3 to 36.4	0.58 to 2.3	0.38 to 1.5	0.63 to 1.56
7 to 10 years	0.18	153	31.5 to 39.4	36.4 to 54.6	0.96 to 3.8	0.63 to 2.5	1.0 to 3.13
Over 10 years	0.18[b]	299[c]	31.5 to 47.2	45.5 to 91.0	0.96 to 3.8	0.63 to 2.5	1.56 to 5.2

[a] 1.6 μmol/kg body weight per day in infants receiving infant formulae only
[b] 0.14 mmol iron supplement in women prior to menopause and a supplement of 0.5–to 1 mmol during pregnancy and lactation
[c] Extra zinc supplement during pregnancy 76 μmol and during lactation 153 μmol

concentrations of each mineral during the first week of lactation (Mendelson *et al.* 1982).

The increasing use of soya-based products and the expanding intake of high phytate fibre-rich foods exposes a large number of the population to the problems related to the availability of trace minerals (see pp.000). The DHSS (1980c) report suggested that meat contributes 36% zinc, 28% copper and 24% iron intake in the UK diet. The decreased consumption of meat because of its expense and the recommendations to decrease saturated fat intake and/or energy intake increases the risk of marginal trace mineral intakes. Hambidge *et al.* (1972) reported growth improvement with zinc supplements in children with marginal zinc intakes from diets with a low meat content.

Marginal deficiency of iron, zinc and vitamin C may predispose an individual to the effect of the chronic exposure to the toxic heavy metals, lead and cadmium, whereas an adequate diet may minimize such exposure and afford some degree of protection (Underwood 1977).

Fluoride from fluoridated water or supplements has been shown to greatly reduce the risk of dental caries (*Lacent*, Editorial 1981). Although excess fluoride is toxic, provided there is 0.07 ppm in water a supplement of 13.2 to 52.6 μmol (0.25 to 1 mg) fluoride per day is appropriate for age and fluoride content of the local water is considered safe and is recommended for children and particularly for those requriing diets containing large or frequent intakes of refined carbohydrate(s).

Therapeutic Diets

The restriction of conventional foods and their replacement with man-made substitutes required in many therapeutic diets result in a reduction in mineral intake and greatly increases the risk of trace mineral deficiencies. The increased losses and poor absorption accompanying conditions such as PEM, cystic fibrosis, protein-losing enteropathy and renal disease, increase the need for trace minerals and such patients are at particular risk of deficiency. Recommendations for supplements are given for specific diets. Further evaluation of these recommendations, the products available and development of new products including milk substitutes and mineral supplements are urgently needed. The risk of interactions and toxicity must also be borne in mind when recommending dietary supplements.

MINERAL SUPPLEMENTS

Mineral supplements currently available fall into 4 categories:

Comprehensive Mineral Mixture

Aminogran Mineral Mixture and Metabolic Mineral Mixture (SHS) contain a range of macro and trace minerals (Table 3.6). Such products are used in severely restricted module diets such as those for inborn errors of protein metabolism, e.g., phenylketonuria and maple syrup urine disease when the protein substitute is not fortified with adequate minerals; in the preparation of module diets for malabsorption based on protein sources such as Comminuted Chicken (Cow & Gate), Maxipro (SHS), Albumaid Complete (SHS); and where natural food is severely restricted such as in 'traditional' ketogenic diets, oligoallergenic diets or low protein diets used in the hyperammonaemias and organic acidaemias. They are contraindicated where an imbalance of minerals would occur because of the contribution of minerals from other sources, e.g., excess sodium intake because of the necessity for sodium bicarbonate to correct acidosis and in chronic renal failure because of their sodium and phosphate content. Care must be taken in their use in infants in order to avoid a high solute intake and/or hyperosmolar feed. Normally for infants each 1 g mineral mixture requires dilution with at least 100 ml fluid and a dose of 1.5 g/kg per day is used under 5.5 kg actual weight. Thereafter a full dose of 8 g per day is adequate or an appropriate intake according to the natural food contribution of the diet. In the older child the mineral mixture can be given as a flavoured medicine in divided doses, with a separate drink.

Trace Mineral Supplement

There is no commercial preparation of trace mineral supplement currently available. A home-made formula has been used for many years at the Hospital for Sick Children, London, and was evaluated by Aggett et al. (1983). The amended formula and its composition is given in Table 3.7. A supplementary dose of 1 to 2 g per day is used in feeds and diets low in trace minerals. The composition is not however considered optimal in the light of current knowledge. New commercial preparations require evaluation before their adequacy can be established.

Table 3.6 Comparison of comprehensive mineral mixtures. (Data from manufacturers 1984.)

100 g	Aminogran Mineral Mixture (Allen & Hanbury Ltd)		Metabolic Mineral Mixture (SHS)		Calcium-free Mineral Mixture (SHS)	
	mmol	g	mmol	g	mmol	g
Calcium	202.5	8.1	204.6	8.2	Nil	Nil
Potassium	212.8	8.3	212.3	8.3	522	20.4
Sodium	173.9	4.0	172.2	3.96	423	9.7
Magnesium	39.9	0.97	39.9	0.97	98	2.4
Chloride	51.3	1.82	50.8	1.8	Nil	Nil
Phosphorus	193.5	6.0	192.4	5.96	473	14.6
Lactate		31.96		32	Nil	Nil
Sulphate		3.96		N/S	N/S	N/S
		mg		mg		mg
Iron	1.1	63	1.1	63	2.78	155
Copper	0.2	13	0.2	13	0.50	32
Zinc	0.7	48	0.7	48	1.79	118
Manganese	0.07	4	0.1	5.7	0.25	14
Iodine	Trace	N/S	0.006	0.76	0.015	1.87
Molybdenum	Trace	N/S	0.0016	0.15	0.0039	0.37
Aluminium	Trace	N/S	0.0007	0.02	0.0017	0.05
Cobalt	Trace	N/S	N/S	N/S	N/S	N/S
Normal dose per day						
Infants	1.5 g/kg to 8 g		1.5 g/kg to 8 g		0.5 g/kg to 4 g	
Children	8g		8g		8g	

Combined Vitamin and Mineral Supplements

A number of preparations for combined vitamin and mineral supplements (see examples in Table 3.2) are available. Cow & Gate Vitamin-Mineral Supplement Tablets (6 to 12 daily) are one of the most comprehensive, Forceval Junior capsules have the advantage of being a one-capsule dose. Adult Seravit, Infant (RD222) and Modified (RD079) Seravit have recently become available from SHS, and may prove useful supplements in some patients once further clinical data on their adequacy is available. These products contain chromium and Infant Seravit also contains selinium.

Inorganic Salts

The inorganic salt of a mineral is frequently less appropriate than the same element in its organic form present in food. However, supplements may be required either prophylactically or in the treatment of actual or potential deficiency. A number of preparations are available and an appropriate dose can be prescribed, e.g.,

1 × Sandocal tablet (Sandoz)	$\simeq$ 400 mg calcium	= 10 mmol elemental calcium
1 g calcium gluconate	= 89.4 mg calcium	= 2.3 mmol elemental calcium
1 × 300 mg calcium lactate tablet	= 39 mg calcium	$\simeq$ 1 mmol elemental calcium
1 × 600 mg calcium lactate tablet	= 78 mg calcium	$\simeq$ 2 mmol elemental calcium
1 g zinc sulphate	= 457 mg zinc	$\simeq$ 7 mmol elemental zinc
1 g zinc acetate	= 600 mg zinc	$\simeq$ 9.2 mmol elemental zinc
220 mg Zincomed capsules (Medo) (zinc sulphate)	= 50 mg zinc	$\simeq$ 0.8 mmol elemental zinc
0.15 ml Endekay (7 drops) (Westone) (0.5 mg sodium fluoride)	= 0.25 mg fluoride	= 13.2 mmol elemental flouride
0.25 mg Zymafluor tablets (Zyma) (sodium fluoride)	= 0.25 mg fluoride	= 13.2 μmol elemental fluoride
1 mg Zymafluor tablets (Zyma)(sodium fluoride)	= 1 mg fluoride	= 52.6 μmol elemental flouride

Specific Inborn Errors of Metabolism Involving Trace Minerals

Occasionally a specific mineral is involved in a particular clinical condition, e.g., zinc supplements are essential in the treatment of acrodermatitis enteropathica (Atherton *et al.* 1979; Aggett 1983), copper in Menke's disease (Camakaris *et al.* 1983), potassium chloride in congenital chloridorrhoea (Milla 1982), phosphate and vitamin D in hypophosphataemic rickets (Hambidge & Walravens

Table 3.7   Supplementary trace mineral mixture (not commercially available).

1 g contains:			
20 mg ferrous sulphate	4.0 mg	iron	= 71.7 μmol
2 mg copper sulphate	0.51 mg	copper	= 8.03 μmol
3.2 mg zinc acetate or 4.2 zinc sulphate	1.92 mg	zinc	= 29.4 μmol
2 mg manganese sulphate	0.49 mg	manganese	= 8.9 μmol
80 μg potassium iodide	61.0 μg	iodine	= 0.48 μmol
	21.5 μg	potassium	= Trace
30 μg potash alum	1.1 μg	aluminum	= 0.04 μmol
30 μg cobalt sulphate	11.3 μg	cobalt	= 0.19 μmol
30 μg sodium molybdate	11.9 μg	molybdenum	= 0.12 μmol
970 mg suitable 'dry powder' filler, e.g. glucose or fructose			

Finely grind and mix, store in an airtight non-metallic container. Normally 1 to 2 g of the mixture is added to the day's feeds and the mixture should not be strained after the addition. The feed should be shaken immediately before use; any coloured specks noted in the feed are due to the trace minerals.

1982), magnesium in primary hypomagnesaemia (Hambidge & Walravens 1982), and currently oral zinc supplements are being used in the management of Wilson's disease which is the best known disorder of copper metabolism and accumulation (Van Caillie-Bertrand *et al.* 1985).

A low nickel diet has been advocated in the treatment of patients with chronic nickel dermatitis (Kaaber *et al.* 1978).

Conclusion

The adequacy of dietary trace mineral intake is related not only to the calculated intake but to a variety of dietary, intestinal and metabolic phenomena which cannot be evaluated precisely. There is therefore a need for vigilance during the management of individual patients and population groups at risk of developing deficiency of trace minerals and for clinical and metabolic assessment of differing dietary therapeutic and synthetic regimens including parenteral nutrition.

REFERENCES

ABUMRAD N. N., SCHNEIDER A. J., STEEL D. & ROGERS L. S. (1981) Amino acid intolerance during prolonged total parenteral nutrition reversed by molybdate therapy. *American Journal of Clinical Nutrition* **34**, 2551–9.

AGGETT P. J. (1983) Acrodermatitis enteropathica. *Journal of Inherited Metabolic Disease* **6** (suppl. I), 39–43.

AGGETT P. J. & HARRIES J. T. (1979) Current status of zinc in health and disease states. *Archives of Disease in Childhood* **54**, 909–17.

AGGETT P. J., ATHERTON D. J., MORE J., DAVEY J., DELVES H. T. & HARRIES J. T. (1980) Symptomatic zinc deficiency in a breast-fed, preterm infant. *Archives of Disease in Childhood* **55**, 547–50.

AGGETT P. J. & DAVIES N. T. (1983) Some nutritional aspects of trace metals. *Journal of Inherited Metabolic Disease* **6** (Suppl. 1), 22–30.

AGGETT P. J., MORE J. M., THORN J. M., DELVES H. T., CORNFIELD M. & CLAYTON B. E. (1983) Evaluation of the trace metal supplements for a synthetic low lactose diet. *Archives of Disease in Childhood* **58**, 433–7.

ALEXANDER F. W., CLAYTON B. E. & DELVES H. T. (1974) Mineral and trace metal balances in children receiving normal and synthetic diets. *Quarterly Journal of Medicine* **43**, 89–111.

ANDERSSON H., NÄVERT B., BINGHAM S. A., ENGLYST H. N. & CUMMINGS J. H. (1983) The effect of breads containing similar amounts of phytate but different amounts of wheat bran on calcium, zinc and iron balance in man. *British Journal of Nutrition* **50**, 503–10.

ATHERTON D. J., MULLER D. P. R., AGGETT P. J. & HARRIES J. T. (1979) A defect in zinc uptake by jejunal biopsies in arcodermatitis enteropathica. *Clinical Science* **56**, 505–7.

BRIGGS M. H. (1973) Fertility and high dose vitamin C. *Lancet* **2**, 1083.

BRIGGS M. H., GARCIA WEBB P. J. & DAVIES P. (1973) Urinary oxalate and Vitamin C supplements. *Lancet* **2**, 201.

BUNKER V. W. & CLAYTON B. E. (1983) Trace element content of commercial enteral feeds. *Lancet* **2**, 426–8.

CAMAKARIS J., PHILLIPS M., DANKS D. M., BROWN R. & STEVENSON T. (1983) Mutations in humans and animals which affect copper metabolism. *Journal of Inherited Metabolic Disease* **6** (Suppl. I), 44–50.

CHANARIN I. (1982) Disorders of vitamin absorption. In Harries J. T. (ed.) *Clinics of Gastroenterology: Familiar Inherited Abnormalities* Volume II, No 1, pp.73–85. Holt Saunders, London.

COCHRANE W. A. (1965) Overnutrition in prenatal & neonatal life: a problem? Symposium on nutrition. *Canadian Medical Association Journal* **93**, No. 17, 895–9.

COUGHLAN, M. (1983) The biological role of molybdenum. *Journal of Inherited Metabolic Disease* **6** (Suppl. I), 70–7.

CUMMINGS J. H., HILL M. J., JIVRAJ T., HOUSTON H., BRANCH W. J. & JENKINS D. J. A. (1979) *American Journal of Clinical Nutrition* **32**, 2086–93.

DAUNCEY M. J., SHAW J. C. L. & URMAN J. (1977) The absorption and retention of magnesium, zinc, copper by low birthweight infants fed pasteurized human breast milk. *Pediatric Research* **11**, 1033–9.

DAVIDSON SIR S., PASSMORE R., BROCK J. F. & TRUSWELL A. S. (1979) *Human Nutrition & Dietetics*, 7th ed. Churchill Livingstone, Edinburgh.

Vitamins and Minerals 145

Davies N.T. (1981) An appraisal of newer trace elements. *Phil. Trans. Royal Society, London* **294**, 171–84.

Davies N. T. (1982) Effects of phytic acid on mineral availability. In Vahouny G. V. & Kritchovsky D. (eds) *Dietary Fibre in Health and Disease*, pp.105–16. Plenum Press, New York.

DHSS (1979) *The Recommended Amounts of Food Energy and Nutrients for Groups of People in the UK*. Report No. 15. HMSO, London.

DHSS (1980a) *Rickets and Osteomalacia*. Report No. 19. HMSO, London.

DHSS (1980b) *Artificial Feeds for the Young Infant*. Report No. 18. HMSO, London.

DHSS (1980c) *Committee on Medical Aspects of Food Policy. Report to the Panel on Novel Foods Which Simulate Meat*. Report of Health and Social Subjects. HMSO, London.

Doisey E. A. (Jr) (1972) Micronutrient controls on biosynthesis of clotting, protein and cholesterol. In Hemphill E. D. (ed) *Trace Substances in Environmental Health VI*, p.193. University of Missouri Press, Columbia.

Ellis R. & Morris E. R. (1981) Relation between phytic acid and trace metals in wheat, bran and soybean. *Cereal Chemistry* **58**, 367–70.

Erdman J. W. (1979) Oilseed phytates: nutritional implications. *Journal of American Oil Chemical Society* **56**, 736–41.

FAO/WHO (1976) *Recommended International Standards for Foods for Infants and Children. Joint FAO/WHO Food Standards Programme*. Codex Alimentarius Commission. FAO, Rome.

Fell G. S., Cuthbertson D. P., Morrison C., Fleck A., Queen K., Bessant R. & Hussain S. L. (1973) Urinary zinc levels as an indication of muscle catabolism. *Lancet* **1**, 280–2.

Fleming C. R., Lie J. T., McCall J. T., O'Brien J. F., Baillie E. E. & Thistle J. L. (1982) Selenium deficiency and fatal cardiomyopathy in a patient on home parenteral nutrition. *Gastroenterology* **83**, 689–93.

Forth W. & Rummel W. (1975) Gastrointestinal absorption of heavy metals. In Forth W. & Rummel W. (eds) *Pharmacology of Intestinal Absorption: Gastrointestinal Absorption of Drugs, Vol. II*, pp.599–746. Pergamon Press, Oxford.

Francis D.E.M. (in press) *Diets for Sick Children*, 4th ed. Blackwell Scientific Publications, London.

Franz K. B., Kennedy B. M. & Fellers D. A. (1980) Relative bioavailability of zinc from selected cereals and legumes using rat growth. *Journal of Nutrition* **110**, 2272–83.

Freund H., Atamian S. & Fischer J. E. (1979) Chromium deficiency during total parenteral nutrition. *Journal of American Medical Association* **241**, 496–8.

Golden M. H. N. & Golden B. E. (1981) Trace elements. Potential importance in human nutrition with particular reference to zinc and vanadium. *British Medical Bulletin* **37**, No. 1, 31–6.

Hambidge K. M. & Walravens P. A. (1982) Disorders of mineral metabolism. In Harries J. T. (ed.) *Clinics in Gastroenterology: Familiar Inherited Abnormalities* Vol. II, No. 1, pp.109–11. W. B. Saunders, London.

HAMBIDGE C., JACOBS M. & BAUM J. D. (1972) Low levels of zinc in hair, anorexia, poor growth and hypogeusia in children. *Pediatric Research* **6**, 868–74.

HARLAND B. F. & PETERSEN M. (1978) Nutritional status of lacto-ovo, vegetarian Trappist monks. *Journal of American Dietetic Association* **72**, 295–64.

HARRELL R. F., CAPP R. H., DAVIS D. R., PEERLESS J. & RAVITZ L. R. (1981) Can nutritional supplements help mentally-retarded children? An exploratory study. *Proceedings of National Academy of Science of the USA* **78**, No. 1 574–8.

HARZER G. & KAUER H. (1982) Binding of zinc to casein. *American Journal of Clinical Nutrition* **35**, 981–7.

HUGHES C., DUTTON S. & TRUSWELL A. S. (1981) High intakes of ascorbic acid and urinary oxalate. *Journal of Human Nutrition* **35**, 274–80.

JAMES W. P. T. (1983) Proposals for Nutritional Guidelines for Health Education in Britain. A discussion paper. National Advisory Committee on Nutrition Education. Health Education Council, London.

JEEJEEBHOY K. N., CHU R. C., MARLISS E. B., GREENBERG G. R. & BRUCE-ROBERTSON A. (1977) Chromium deficiency, glucose intolerance, and neuropathy reversed by chromium supplementation in a patient receiving long-term total parenteral nutrition. *American Journal of Clinical Nutrition* **30**, 531–8.

KAABER K., VEREIN N. K. & TJELL J. C. (1978) Low nickel diet in the treatment of patients with chronic nickel dermatitis. *British Journal of Dermatology* **98**, 197.

KARPEL J. T. & PEDAN V. H. (1972) Copper deficiency in long-term parenteral nutrition. *Journal of Pediatrics* **80**, 32–6.

KAY R. G., TASMAN-JONES C., PYBUS J., WHITING R. & BLACK H. (1976) A syndrome of acute zinc deficiency during total parenteral alimentation in man. *Annals of Surgery* **183**, 331–340.

Lancet, Editorial (1981) Dental caries and fluoride. *Lancet* **1**, 1351.

Lancet, Editorial (1983) Selenium perspective. *Lancet* **1**, 685.

LAWSON M. S., CLAYTON B. E., DELVES H. T. & MITCHELL J. D. (1977) Evaluation of a new mineral and trace metal supplement for use with synthetic diets. *Archives of Diseases in Childhood* **52**, 62–7.

LOMBECK I. (1983) Evaluation of selenium states in children. *Journal of Inherited Metabolic Disease* **6** (Suppl. 1) 83–4.

LOMBECK I., EBERT K.H., KASPEREK K., FEINENDEGEN L.E. & BREMER H.J. (1984) Selenium intake of infants and young children, healthy children and dietetically treated patients with Phenylketonuria. *European Journal of Paediatrics* **143**, 199–202.

McLAREN D. S. (1982) Vitamin deficiency, toxicity and dependency. In

Burman D. & McLaren D. S. (eds) *Textbook of Paediatric Nutrition,* 2nd ed., pp.143–63. Churchill Livingstone, Edinburgh.

McLaren D. S. & Burman D. (eds) (1982) *Textbook of Paediatric Nutrition,* 2nd ed. Churchill Livingstone, Edinburgh.

McMillan J. A., Landow S. A. & Oski F. A. (1976) Iron sufficiency in breast fed infants and the availability of iron from human milk. *Pediatrics* **58,** 686–91.

Mann T. P., Wilson K. M. & Clayton B. E. (1965) A deficiency state in infants on synthetic foods. *Archives of Disease in Childhood* **40,** 364–75.

Mendelson R. A., Anderson G. H. & Bryan M. H. (1982) Zinc, copper and iron content of milk from mothers of preterm and full-term infants (1982). *Early Human Development* **6,** 145–151.

Mendelson R. A., Bryan M. H. & Anderson G. H. (1983) Trace mineral balances in preterm infants fed their own mother's milk. *Journal of Pediatric Gastroenterology & Nutrition* **2,** 256–61.

Milla P. (1982) Disorders of electrolyte absorption. In Harries J. T. (ed.) *Clinics in Gastroenterology. Familiar Inherited Abnormalities* Vol 11, No 1, pp.37–42. Saunders, London.

Muller D. P. R., Lloyd J. K. & Bird A. C. (1977) Long-term management of abetalipoproteinaernia. Possible role of vitamin E. *Archives of Disease in Childhood* **52,** 209–14.

National Research Council (1980) *Food and Nutrition Board Recommended Dietary Allowances,* 9th revised edn. National Academy of Sciences, Washington DC.

Nestlé (in press) *Trace Minerals* 8th Nestlé Nutrition Workshop. Chairman R. Chandra Munich.

O'Dell B. L. (1979) Effect of soy protein on trace mineral availability. In Wilche *et al.* (ed.) *Soy Protein and Human Nutrition,* pp.187–207. Academic Press, London.

Reinhold J. G., Faradji B., Abad P. & Ismail-Beigi F. (1976) Decreased absorption of calcium, magnesium, zinc and phosphorus by humans due to increased fibre and phosphorus consumption as wheat bread. *Journal of Nutrition* **106,** (4) 493–503.

Rhead W. J. & Schrauzer G. N. (1971) Risks of long-term ascorbic acid over dosage. *Nutritional Reviews* **29,** 262–3.

Saner G. (1980) *Chromium in Nutrition and Disease.* A. R. Liss Inc., New York.

Smith, G. F., Spiker D., Peterson C., Cicchetti D. & Justice P. (1983) Failure of vitamin/mineral supplementation in Down's syndrome. Letter, *Lancet* July 2, 2, 8340:41.

Thorn J. M., Aggett, P. J., Delves H. T. & Clayton B. E. (1978) Mineral and trace metal supplement for use with synthetic diets based on comminuted chicken. *Archives of Disease in Childhood* **53,** 931–8.

Tripp J. H., Francis D. E. M., Knight J. A. & Harries J. T. (1979) Infant feeding practices: a cause of concern. *British Medical Journal* **2,** 707–709.

UNDERWOOD E. J. (1977) *Trace Elements in Human and Animal Nutrition*, 4th ed. Academic Press, London.

UNDERWOOD E. J. (1981) Trace metals in human and animal health. *Journal of Human Nutrition* **35**, 37–48.

VALLEE B. L. (1983) A role for zinc and gene expression. *Journal of Inherited Metabolic Disease* **6** (Suppl. I) 31–3.

VAN CAILLIE-BERTRAND M., DEGENHART H.J., VISSER H.K.A., SINAASAPPEL M. & BOUQUET J. (1985) Oral zinc sulphate for Wilson's disease. *Archives of Disease in Childhood* **60**, 656–9.

WADMAN S. K. (1983) Inborn error of molybdenum cofactor deficiency. *Journal of Inherited Metabolic Disease* **6** (Suppl. I), 78–83.

WALKER A. P. R. (1951) Cereals, phytic acid and calcification. *Lancet* **2**, 244–8.

WILLIAMS A. F. & BAUM J. D. (eds) (1984) *Human Milk Banking*. Nestlé Nutrition Workshop Series, Vol 5, Raven, New York.

WISE A. (1983) Dietary factors determining the biological activities of phytate. *Nutrition Abstracts and Reviews in Clinical Nutrition*. Series A, Vol 53, No 9, 791–806.

WHO (1973) *Trace Elements in Human Nutrition*. Technical Report Series No. 532. WHO, Geneva.

ZIMMERMAN A. W., HAMBIDGE M., LEPOW M. L., GREENBERG R. D., STOVER M. L. & CASEY C. E. (1982) Acrodermatitis in breastfed premature infants: evidence for a defect of mammary zinc secretion. *Pediatrics* **69**, 176–83.

APPENDIX 1

Borderline Substances

In the UK a number of proprietary foods used in treatment are classified as drugs for certain conditions. The Secretary of State for Social Services has appointed a committee to advise where particular preparations should be regarded as drugs and their recommendations are published as an appendix in each edition of the *British National Formulary, Drug Tariff* and *MIMS*. Prescription form FC 10, used for prescribing such products, should be marked ACBS where the item prescribed is listed for the condition concerned.

REFERENCES

BRITISH NATIONAL FORMULARY. British Medical Association and The Pharmaceutical Society of Great Britain. Pitman Press, Bath.
DRUG TARIFF. Prepared under Regulation 28 of the National Health Service (General Medical and Pharmaceutical Services). Regulation 1974, Family Practitioner Services Division 2C1, Elephant and Castle, London.
MIMS. Medical Publications Ltd, London.

APPENDIX 2

SI Units Used in Nutrition

CONVERSION FOR ENERGY

Conversion of kilojoules (kJ) to kilocalories (kcal)

kJ	kcal
9000	2151
8000	1912
7000	1673
6000	1434
5000	1195
4000	956
3500	837
3000	717
2500	600
2000	478
1500	359
1000[a]	239
500	120
100	24
1	0.239

[a] 1 megajoule (MJ).
1 kcal = 4.184 kJ.

Units of energy from different food types

	kJ	kcal
1 g Protein	17	4
1 g Fat	37	9
1 g Carbohydrate	16	4
1 g Alcohol	29	7

Appendix 2

CONVERSION FOR MINERALS

Calcium	$\dfrac{mg}{40.0}$	
Chloride	$\dfrac{mg}{35.5}$	
Copper	$\dfrac{mg}{63.6}$	
Iodine	$\dfrac{mg}{126.9}$	
Iron	$\dfrac{mg}{55.8}$	millimole (mmol)
Magnesium	$\dfrac{mg}{24.0}$	
Phosphorus	$\dfrac{mg}{31.0}$	
Potassium	$\dfrac{mg}{39.0}$	
Sodium	$\dfrac{mg}{23.0}$	
Zinc	$\dfrac{mg}{65.4}$	

VITAMINS

Vitamin D_3 1 µg = 40.0 IU
             1 IU = 0.025 µg

Vitamin A   1 µg = 3.3 IU retinol (Vitamin A_1 alcohol)
             1 IU = 0.30 µg retinol (Vitamin A_1 alcohol)
             1 IU = 0.60 µg carotene

Conversion for General Measurements

Oven temperatures

Fahrenheit (°F)	Celsius (°C)	Gas Regulo Number	
175	80		
200	100		cool
225	110		slow
250	120	½	
275	140	1	
300	150	2	
325	160	3	moderate
350	180	4	
375	190	5	fairly hot
400	200	6	
425	220	7	hot
450	230	8	
475	240	9	very hot
500	260		
525	270		

Approximate metric conversion

1 ounce (oz) = 28.4 gramme (g) or millilitre (ml) or cubic centimetre (cc)
1 pound (lb) = 450 g
2.2 lb = 1000 g = 1 kilogram (kg)
1 pint = 20 ounces = 560 millilitres (ml)

100 g or ml = 3½ oz
200 g or ml = 7 oz
30 g or ml approximately = 1 oz
1000 g or ml = 35 oz

2.54 centimetres (cm) = 1 inch
100 cm = 1 metre = 39″
12″ = 30.5 cm

Volumetric measurements

	ml
Standard 8 oz cup	240
Standard teaspoon	5
Standard tablespoon	15

Scales for Use with Weighed Diets

A simple accurate diet scale which is robust and easy to use with digital reading or a clear dial is now easier to obtain. I have found the clock dial or digital scale with 5 g and ¼ oz increments satisfactory for home use, as even children can manage this type, and the accuracy is satisfactory for diets such as described in this book.

For hospital kitchens, there are many types of metric scales available covering a wide range of accuracy and cost. Increments of 1 g are suitable for most purposes. Those with a tare mechanism enable the weight of the container in which the food is weighed to be counteracted. The ingredients of special infant feeds may need to be weighed, but because of the need for aseptic preparation the scale pans should be sterilizable or the ingredients weighed into sterilized jugs on scales with a tare mechanism.

Index

Note Page numbers in *italics* refer to those pages on which tables appear.

155